ROUTLEDGE LIBRARY EDITIONS: HEALTH, DISEASE & SOCIETY

Volume 1

# HEALTH CARE OF THE ELDERLY

# HEALTH CARE OF THE ELDERLY

## Essays in Old Age Medicine, Psychiatry and Services

Edited by
TOM ARIE

Routledge
Taylor & Francis Group
LONDON AND NEW YORK

First published in 1981 by Croom Helm Ltd.

This edition first published in 2022
by Routledge
4 Park Square, Milton Park, Abingdon, Oxon OX14 4RN

and by Routledge
605 Third Avenue, New York, NY 10158

*Routledge is an imprint of the Taylor & Francis Group, an informa business*



*British Library Cataloguing in Publication Data*
A catalogue record for this book is available from the British Library

ISBN: 978-0-367-52469-2 (Set)
ISBN: 978-1-032-25761-7 (Volume 1) (hbk)
ISBN: 978-1-032-25769-3 (Volume 1) (pbk)
ISBN: 978-1-003-28491-8 (Volume 1) (ebk)

DOI: 10.4324/9781003284918

**Publisher's Note**
The publisher has gone to great lengths to ensure the quality of this reprint but points out that some imperfections in the original copies may be apparent.

**Disclaimer**
The publisher has made every effort to trace copyright holders and would welcome correspondence from those they have been unable to trace.

# Health Care of the Elderly

ESSAYS IN OLD AGE MEDICINE,
PSYCHIATRY AND SERVICES

EDITED BY TOM ARIE

CROOM HELM LONDON

Croom Helm Ltd, 2-10 St John's Road, London SW11

British Library Cataloguing in Publication Data

Health care of the elderly.
1. Aged - Care and hygiene
I. Arie, Tom
362.6 HV1451

ISBN 0-7099-0252-2

Printed in Great Britain by
Redwood Burn Limited
Trowbridge and Esher

# CONTENTS

# FIGURES AND TABLES

## Figures



## Tables

# PREFACE

Contributors to this book were asked to write a personal essay – rather than a conventional review, or a report of work done. Professional literature abounds with each of the latter, whilst essays these days are rarer.

Contributors were told that the emphasis should be on ideas. They were asked to step back from detailed data, using them to support ideas rather than reporting them for their own sake. In inviting the contributions, I wrote, 'I hope that people may see this as an opportunity to write something that they will enjoy writing, and which a fairly wide range of (not necessarily technically sophisticated) readers will enjoy reading; and that they will be able to consider some of the things which may have been edged out by space, comprehensiveness or other constraints in more conventional contributions.'

Most of the contributions are from people eminent in their field, though there are included a few pieces by bright younger people, all of whom have already contributed enough to our field to make their future eminence safely worth betting on. The style in which they have responded to my invitation to write an essay rather than a wholly formal piece varies from one to another, as one might expect; but in the writing of all of them, as in the editing, the main concern has been to catch the reader's interest. This aims to be an unstuffy book on very serious matters.

Tom Arie
Nottingham

# 1 INTRODUCTION. HEALTH CARE OF THE *VERY* ELDERLY: TOO FRAIL A BASKET FOR SO MANY EGGS?

Tom Arie

'Health Care of the Elderly' is the name of our department in Nottingham. This book's contributors come from much further afield than just our own department, but a brief word about our department is appropriate, for from it this book takes both its name and its joint approach. The care of the elderly is nothing if it is not a collaborative enterprise. We in Nottingham have tried to go further, by constructing a joint department comprising physicians, psychiatrists and other health workers concerned with the elderly. In short, we have moved from collaboration to unity. I hope that the book will be seen to express the unity of the health care of the elderly.

In Nottingham we each 'do our own thing'; psychiatrists practice psychiatry and physicians medicine. But we have a common identity and allegiance, we share facilities (including, importantly, a joint building) and much of our nascent research is joint. Supporting our patients and their families is our main business, for our joint approach attempts to ensure that they neither fall between different professions and services, nor get bounced from one to another; but we are very much aware that alongside support for our patients, we have an important job to do in supporting each other.

So we have made a start in making a unity of services for the elderly. We have a long way to go, but already it is clear that this style works, and we enjoy working in this way. Together we serve a defined population in which our services are available to help any old person. There is nothing selective about our clientele: or rather, we do not select them and if there is bias, it is towards the very aged and very infirm. For these are our people: the very aged with multiple infirmities and often with failing brains. Of course, we see many 'younger' old people and many with more straightforward medical or psychiatric problems; but at the centre of our concerns are the very infirm elderly. It might be more appropriate to describe our work as the Health Care of the Very Elderly.

**The Novel Commonplaceness of Extreme Old Age**

It is, of course, the very aged whose numbers are increasing most rapidly in our country, and in most countries similar to our own. It is in them that the now well documented conjunction of physical, mental and social privations is at its most intense; and the most damaging of all these, dementia, rises sharply in its incidence over the age of 80, affecting about one in five of the population of that age. One in five means that four out of five very aged people are *not* demented, but dementia raises the most taxing issues of medical care, and the most expensive ones – for it is the greatest generator of breakdown, of demand for institutional care and of family burden and crisis. David Jolley and I have together written on these matters on several occasions, and in his chapter in this book he sets out the scale of this problem, which promises to be the biggest challenge to health and social services in all developed countries for the foreseeable future; and he presents approaches which have been shown to work. Kenneth Shulman, also a former colleague, is developing a similar service in Toronto – and in part because of the way care is organised there, in part because of the familiar operation of the 'Inverse Care Law', he is seeing far fewer demented patients than patients with functional disorders – a state of affairs which, as he says, he intends to change.

In our teaching we constantly focus on the very aged. The University of Nottingham has provided a full-time attachment of one month's duration to our department for all medical students; during this time they have an 'apprenticeship' to the services of the department, a formal course of teaching, and an opportunity to tackle a particular topic in some depth. We see it as a special responsibility to put this attachment to good use (few medical courses provide as much time for teaching the care of the elderly). We therefore take special pains to avoid merely duplicating the teaching of other departments in medicine and psychiatry, but constantly seek to emphasise the special issues that arise in the elderly. This book should illustrate both the fascination and scientific interest of these matters, and the barriers which stand between old people and effective medical care. Norman Exton-Smith's chapter illustrates well what have been called 'the vicious circles of social medicine' – in this case, the association of maximum biological risk with maximum social disadvantage. Such vicious circles pervade the care of the very aged, and illustrations abound in Grimley Evans's chapter and, in rather different ways, in Donald Calne's.

Very aged people get a poor deal from services; and not all the services which we disburse, often enthusiastically and almost always expensively, have been shown to be effective. Graham Mulley reviews attempts to measure the effectiveness of our rehabilitative services in relation to strokes; James Williamson looks at the value of screening and surveillance, whilst Olive Stevenson attempts both to define the particular task of the social worker in relation to aged people, and to consider some of the reasons why this task is so often not fulfilled. Roy Boyd, from a different point of view, makes an attempt to give precision to, and to make sense of, that often woolly and overworked category, the 'social problem'.

Nor, as Klaus Bergmann and Felix Post show, are the elderly, and the very elderly, by any means immune from functional mental disorder, often of an eminently treatable kind. Only in recent decades has the importance of affective disorder in old people come to be widely recognised, with massively beneficial consequences for old people, who formerly were too often relegated to the category of the 'senile' and thus hopeless. Similarly, the scale of neurotic disorder and maladjustment in old people, including the very old, is now recognised (by contrast with the former comfortable assumption that emotional turbulence becomes extinct with ageing, 'all passion spent'). This growing clinical and epidemiological understanding, in which Post and Bergmann have been among the pioneers, has already made successful contributions to a rational basis both for treatment and for the planning of services. And such knowledge has also underpinned with facts the debate on the pros and cons of specialised services for very old people which Bernard Isaacs sets out.

I asked Adrian Verwoerdt to write on psychotherapy for the elderly for two reasons: first, because too few people are attempting to think through the issues, such as the ways in which classical psychoanalytic teaching may need to be modified in relation to the elderly, and the scope and limitations of psychotherapy in old people with failing brains. Second, since most psychiatrists who work specially with the elderly are of an empirical disposition, I thought it would be nicely complementary to include a contribution which takes much of its strength from a particiular theoretical framework.

But there is another sense in which the subject of psychotherapy with the very aged is important. For experience with it gives the lie to any impression that the very aged are necessarily without inner turmoil and suffering, or indeed without those dynamics of the psyche which are evident in younger people. The existence of an active inner life in the very old is often implicitly questioned, especially perhaps by those so close to them that the truth could be hard to endure. More light has often been shed on this matter by writers than by clinicians, and in our department we recommend our students to read novels about old people during their period of attachment (and the fact that they take our advice is attested by the constant disappearance of most of these from our library!). Such works include Nell Dunn and Adrian Henri's love story *I Want*, Paul Bailey's *At the Jerusalem*, a delicate and terrifying account of an old lady's life in an old people's home, and that wonderfully restrained picture of two old people's relationship which is Vita Sackville-West's *All Passion Spent*. Simone de Beauvoir's book on old age, though not a novel, yet has the power (and bitterness) of a work by a novelist herself grown old.

But here I want to draw briefly on two sources, each of them reporting what very old people themselves tell us. It is common to distance ourselves from the very old, to assume they don't know, they don't notice, they don't suffer (indeed, that they don't hear, for we often assume they are deaf).

Some months ago, following a BBC programme to do with bereavement, the producer received a letter which he passed on to me. I quote most of it here, with the writer's permission:

Dear Producer,

*Bereavement*

I missed the first 15 minutes of your last programme but, from what I did hear, you appear to have missed the most poignant cases of bereavement – where it touches the old and the very old. No one seems to want to know about them and assumes that only the middle-aged are involved. The lot of the really old is much worse. I am 81 and 2 years ago my wife, then 77, died. The last 2 years have been very hard to bear. I fell in love with her when I was only 20 and she 18. We were married 4 years later and had 54 years of wonderful life together. The only comfort I am offered is that I must have many happy memories. But that is common to all age bereavement. The younger generation can reconstruct their lives, but at 80, no one can see any use for you and you are expected to retire to the corner of a geriatric ward or home. My home – my wife's home – means everything to me – I would hate to leave it.

***

I have a good son and a good daughter and good grandchildren.

> They would never let me suffer physically but nothing they can do can ease my grief of losing my life-long beloved wife. I happen to be fairly active mentally and physically but, even then, life is now a very empty thing. I receive many kindnesses but can do little in return. I am no longer a useful member of the community – that hurts.
>
> Yours sincerely,

It would be absurd to do more than to let these words stand by themselves. The last two sentences sum up much of the predicament of the very elderly in our society – 'I receive many kindnesses but can do little in return. I am no longer a useful member of the community – that hurts.' But there is no escaping the other terrible conclusion of this letter – that even in extreme old age those passions and griefs that we take for granted in younger people, but which we so readily deny in the elderly, are there, and there are fewer distractions or consolations.

This was much in my mind when I was asked to speak recently at a meeting of students on 'Death and the Doctor'. I asked myself why I in particular had been invited, as someone whose work is with the elderly, for it is generally assumed that both death, and bereavement, are gentler when they come to the very old than in the prime of life. Certainly, there is support for this impression from studies of dying people by workers such as John Hinton on the distress of the dying, and by Colin Murray Parkes and many others on the excess morbidity and premature death which may follow bereavement, and which are both commoner in younger people. But that letter reminds us that relative frequency between groups tells us little about the experience of individuals, and that age extinguishes neither sensibilities nor suffering.

Part of my second illustration is a poem. Robert Graves has said that the essence of good poetry is that it says what it has to say in so few words that one would save little money by turning it into a telegram. I am not sure how well this poem by Walter de la Mare stands up to Graves's test, but it is moving and eloquent, and it comes in a passage which I have taken from Ronald Blythe's splendid new book about old age, *The View in Winter*. An 84-year-old schoolmaster is speaking, and Blythe has recorded the interview:

> Old age doesn't necessarily mean that one is entirely old – all old, if you follow me. It doesn't mean that for many people, which is why it is so very difficult. It is complicated by the retention of a lot of

one's youth in an old body. I tend to look upon other old men as old men – and not include myself. It is not vanity; it is just that it is still natural for me to be young in some respects. What is generally assumed to have happened to a man in his eighties has not happened to me. The generalisations which go with my age don't apply. Yet I resent it all in some ways, this being very old, yes, I resent it. I have lost most of my physical strength, and once I was strong and loved doing physical work. I am not used to the loss of my strength and I object when many tasks show that they are now beyond me. I cannot quite believe that I can't carry this or turn, or hold the other. This old part of me worries the young part of me. It could be that it would be better to be all old. I think that De la Mare's got the confusion in a nutshell. His poem, 'A Portrait', says it all. I read it often now and find that the cap fits. Here it is:

Old: yet unchanged; still pottering in his thoughts;
Still eagerly enslaved by books and print;
Less plagued, perhaps, by rigid musts and oughts,
But no less frantic in vain argument:

Punctual at meals; a spendthrift, close as Scot;
Rebellious, tractable, childish – long gone grey!
Impatient, volatile, tongue wearying not –
Loose, too; which, yet, thank heaven, was taught to pray:

'Childish' indeed! a waif on shingle shelf
Fronting the rippled sands, the sun, the sea;
And nought but his marooned precarious self
For questing consciousness and will to be:

To frail a basket for so many eggs –
Loose-woven; gosling? cygnet? Laugh or weep?
Or is the cup at richest in its dregs?
The actual realest on the verge of sleep?

A foolish, fond old man, his bed-time nigh,
Who still at western window stays to win
A transient respite from the latening sky,
And scarce can bear it when the sun goes in.[1]

I want to linger for a moment on one line: 'Too frail a basket for so many eggs'. The image is of a fragile, precarious, inadequate container for a multitude of things themselves fragile – eggs are the symbol of brittleness and fragility. In extreme old age, the inner life may be teeming – 'so *many* eggs' – rather than inert or quiet. Eggs betoken pregnancy, they promise the unfulfilled that which is yet to be; but in everyday life most eggs have their promise aborted: they will be consumed, they won't ever hatch! 'I *resent* it all . . . this being very old,' says Blythe's old schoolmaster; in Dylan Thomas's words, he will 'not go gentle into that good night', but rather will 'rage against the dying of the light' – a famous phrase which echoes that of the present poem: he 'scarce can bear it when the sun goes in'.

Well, it is very old people like this for whom services for the health care of the elderly exist; and 'Too frail a basket for so many eggs' might itself stand as a gloss on those services, which seem unlikely ever, anywhere, to cope adequately with the spiral of expectations. These expectations themselves derive from those very features of modern societies which have extended the life-span and made extreme old age, for the first time in the history of mankind, commonplace.

## Building Confidence

The contributors to this book illuminate with ideas and information the nature and scale of the issues of health, sickness and care of old people which modern industrial (and not only industrial) societies must tackle. They are largely new problems and no previous society can provide parallels or solutions; we have to work them out ourselves. And we must remember that the impact of unprecedented numbers of very aged people raises different issues for different groups: first, there are the old people themselves and the question of what *they* need from society; then there is society as a whole, and the challenge posed by the vast increase in the number (and proportion) of people of pensionable age; then the families and the other 'non-professional' people who provide the bulk of direct support and care; and finally (and often forgotten, though they are a subject of special interest to me), there are the staff who man the services for the elderly. Health services must consider the needs of each of these 'constituencies', balancing them and often compromising, for the perceived interests of any one of these groups do not necessarily point in the same direction as those of all the others.

We believe that the effectiveness of services depends on building confidence – confidence on the part of the local community, confidence among colleagues, confidence among one's own staff. Without such confidence in it even a service which is amply endowed with staff and facilities (and I doubt if there are any such services) will be overwhelmed by escalating demands. But confidence in what? Certainly not in the ability of the service to solve every problem, or to make available whatever resource is perceived as necessary by those who are calling for help. Confidence must be in the service's willingness to respond to any problem that is legitimately in its province, urgently if necessary, and to listen, to understand, and to do its best; to honour its undertakings, and to think again when problems change or solutions are not working. Above all, perhaps, confidence that the service will not let people down when there is real trouble – for many excess demands and 'crises' are testings of the service, or expressions of lack of confidence that it will take notice when a real crisis comes. It is the universal experience of good services which have gained the confidence of those they serve that the 'crises' abate, and that people (colleagues and clients alike) largely stop inflating their demands, in the knowledge that the service will respond and will do its honest best.

We who plan services are constantly preoccupied with issues such as these, but among the many pressures that bear upon us, the voice of old people themselves is heard neither often enough nor loudly enough. America's 'Grey Panthers' may be beginning to change that; but least heard of all are the voices of individual old people such as I have quoted, and their eloquence will, I hope, complement the professional perspective of this book.

Most of this book's contributors are doctors, yet their contributions themselves make clear how much the health care of the elderly depends on non-medical people. I should like to make a final comment on the responsibility of doctors in relation to old people. It would be foolish and dangerous for doctors to collude in 'medicalisation' of all the problems of the elderly. Doctors, I think, are less likely to grab these problems as exclusively their own than is society to find it convenient to assign to a particular profession problems which have no clear solutions: Ivan Illich seems largely to have missed the point that it is much more society's convenience that 'medicalises' complex problems than the avidity of the medical profession to take responsibility for them. And yet medicine does have a unique role in regard to the elderly and it is as well, in introducing a book on the *health* care of the elderly, to remind ourselves of some of the reasons why this is so.

First, of course, is the high incidence of frank medical problems in old people, mostly chronic degenerative conditions and their acute manifestations. Fifty per cent of over-65-year-olds in Britain report lasting chronic sickness, and the elderly have the highest consultation rate of all age groups in general practice, and the highest admission rates to hospitals. Half of all British hospital beds are occupied by the elderly. A recent survey conducted by Age Concern in England found that, at the age of 75 and over, the average person was troubled by six different ailments, many of them seriously limiting. Only 10 per cent of over-75s reported no such ailments.

For the very aged, ill health is an ever present threat. When we are young and things are not going well, we are apt to say, 'Well, at least I have my good health,' rightly expecting that this state of affairs will endure. In old age, a fall, a chill, a small injury may quickly result not only in incapacity, but in loss of independence and choice. By his power to intervene effectively, and when possible to prevent, the doctor has a quite special responsibility in maintaining the health of old people and thus protecting them against those social disabilities of which broken health is often the main cause.

And we have evidence from old people themselves that their main anxiety is about health – greater even than fears of loneliness or financial problems (despite the fact that even in most prosperous countries old people are the biggest group of the poor, and that of the very aged nearly half live alone). Enquiries among old people (such as Audrey Hunt's on behalf of our government's Social Survey) confirm the central importance to them of their health. The maintenance and improvement of the health of their old people is certainly only one part of the complex responses which the unprecedented number of very aged citizens demands from modern societies; but there is no more important, and no more potentially beneficent response.

## Note

1. Ronald Blythe, *The View in Winter* (Allen Lane, London, 1979), p. 226. Copyright © Ronald Blythe, 1979. Reprinted by permission of Penguin Books Ltd. Part of 'A Portrait' by Walter de la Mare reproduced with the permission of The Literary Trustees of Walter de la Mare and The Society of Authors as their representative.

# PART ONE: MEDICINE

# 2 STROKE REHABILITATION: WHAT ARE WE ALL DOING?

Graham Mulley

'Apoplexy is almost restricted to the afternoon of life, a period attended by degeneration of the vascular tunics.'[1]

It has been known since the days of the Hippocratic writers that stroke predominantly affects the elderly. At present, 70 per cent of stroke victims are over 65 years of age. Consequently, much of a geriatric physician's time is spent dealing with the impact of stroke on the individual and his family. Although stroke is very common, we know very little about the best ways of dealing with it.

The best stroke care must combine science with humanity. Only by asking basic questions about what we are doing can we hope to improve management and interest other people in stroke rehabilitation. But life is larger than logic and we must not become so besotted with scientific medicine that we lose sight of the immense value of the human element – the interest and concern, the respect and kindness which our patients need beyond their physical requirements. While it is important, therefore, to assess the scientific value of different forms of treatment, we must be prepared to accept that concepts such as morale and motivation, which are difficult to define and impossible to measure, probably play a crucial role in the healing process.

There are three components of stroke treatment: prevention, acute management and rehabilitation. Stroke prevention is all-important, but much work is needed to put existing knowledge into practice (particularly in the field of blood pressure control) and to discover new ways of preventing stroke. We know little about stroke prevention in the elderly: the efficacy of treatment for lowering blood pressure in old people has yet to be determined; and we do not know the benefit conferred by anticoagulants on symptomless old people with atrial fibrillation. Both primary and secondary prevention are therefore based more on the whim of the doctor than on hard fact.

Acute management of stroke involves specific medical or surgical measures intended to improve the function of the injured area of brain; and the prevention and treatment of complications. For centuries, many agents have been advocated for acute stroke. Medieval physicians applied cautery to the vertex or occiput. In the eighteenth century, treatment of apoplexy was conducted in accordance with stipulated and undeviating precepts: blood was abstracted, drastics (powerful purgatives) were administered together with enemata, emetics and the application of cold to the head. In order to arouse the flagging motion of the animal spirits, patients were given errhines (such as snuff, to cause sneezing), volatile salts and vinegar.[1] In more recent years, a number of drugs have been given in attempts to improve cerebral metabolism. None has been shown to be of practical benefit to the patient. Recently it has been found that reducing the haematocrit may improve cerebral blood flow.[2] It may be that venesection (an 'inconsiderate practice which has proved on the whole more harmful than salutary'[1]) is destined for renaissance.

Although more work must be done in trying to improve brain function in acute stroke, there is much room for improving basic care – prevention of bedsores and contractures, treatment of deep vein thrombosis and chest infection, attention to bowels and bladder, care in handling the hemiplegic shoulder and imagination in communicating with the dysphasic patient.

The lack of effective therapy in acute stroke, despite years of research, may be a contributory factor to the nihilistic attitude towards stroke which is prevalent among many doctors. Certainly there is a marked lack of interest in stroke rehabilitation, which is often considered to be something that other people do when the doctor has become therapeutically bankrupt. It is often thought of as basket-making, strengthening exercises or diversional therapy. Some question the whole basis of rehabilitation: it has been described as a silly euphemism,[3] and the suggestion has been made that the patients should not be subject to unwanted activity but be left in peace to die in dignity. The paucity of firm evidence that rehabilitation is of measurable value has reinforced the general feeling of scepticism and negativism.

In 1888, Gowers wrote:

> The tendency to improvement, by cerebral compensation and by spontaneous disappearance of indirect symptoms, is very marked and it makes it difficult to estimate the actual influence of treatment that is employed. At the same time it renders these cases a tempting field for the assumptions of the quasi-therapist.[4]

In evaluating techniques of rehabilitation, we need to ask fundamental questions which may cause discomfort to those who have an emotional investment in particular forms of treatment: how much recovery would take place without any therapy whatsoever? Are certain practices actually harmful? If treatment is beneficial, must it be performed by a trained professional or would an untrained or partly trained person do the job as effectively? Can we identify which patients are going to benefit from therapy? If so, do we know how and what kind of therapy to give, over how long a period? Should rehabilitation take place in hospital, at home, or elsewhere? What should we do for the stroke patient and his family once active rehabilitation measures stop? And are we certain that those aspects of rehabilitation which interest the professionals are the ones which are of most concern to the patient?

One of the important tenets of geriatric medicine is that multidisciplinary team work is of central importance in successful patient care. As organiser of the team, the doctor must be conversant with the skills of each team member. If we are to improve the management of the stroke patient, we need to examine the role of every member of the team and ascertain what they are trying to do, what they are actually doing, and if there are better ways of doing it. Let us then take a hard look at each individual's role in the rehabilitation of elderly stroke victims.

## The Physiotherapist

There are two components of stroke physiotherapy: preventing or minimising those factors which inhibit recovery of useful movement and encouraging the restoration of function. Rehabilitation is not putting in something which is not there: it is directing and capitalising on the spontaneous recovery which occurs in most stroke patients.

Before the profession of physiotherapy existed, emphasis was placed on the prevention of complications.[5] Nurses were encouraged to perform passive movements early, during the flaccid stage of hemiplegia, in order to keep the joints mobile, prevent muscular contractions and improve the circulation in the limbs. They were also instructed in the importance of turning and positioning of patients. Massage was recommended, which was intended to maintain a flow of sensory impulses and which appeared to reduce spasticity. In addition to physical measures, the importance of sustaining the patient's morale and motivation was emphasised. Coulter[6] wrote that 'the patient should be told that the nurses can only prevent the formation of adhesions and contractures and that the return of movements depends on the patient's efforts'. Later, stress was laid on the importance of the physiotherapist's efforts in sustaining the patient's continued co-operation and motivation which are so necessary for recovery.[7]

As physiotherapy evolved, techniques which had been developed for patients with tabes, polio, cerebral palsy and other neuromuscular disorders were adapted for hemiplegic stroke patients. The aims of treatment were to encourage early walking and restore function by promoting the use of the unaffected side, in addition to preventing deformities and treating those deformities that did occur. In order to discharge the patient from hospital as soon as possible, exercises to strengthen the sound side were supplemented by the use of calipers, tripods and other aids and appliances. These traditional methods of physiotherapy may have succeeded in getting people out of hospital quickly, but the early mobility was achieved at a high cost. The patient usually developed the typical hemiplegic posture: a useless, spastic adducted arm, retracted and depressed at the shoulder, flexed and pronated at the elbow and wrist, with the fist being tightly clenched; a stiff leg with the hip in external rotation, the knee held in extension and the foot plantar flexed. The good arm had to be used primarily to maintain the upright posture and could not be used for other activities. The patient's gait was abnormal: he had to circumduct the leg, and it was very hard work to walk when one half of the body was spastic. Stroke patients tend to fall more often than other people. They usually fall to the affected side, and are unable to use the arm to break the fall. The long bones on the affected side become particularly osteoporotic, and the heavy fall may result in hip fracture.[9] Moreover, the fear of falls is thought to increase spasticity, which may increase the likelihood of falls. In addition to the potential danger produced by the abnormal gait, the spastic walking pattern was readily apparent to everyone and marked out the patient as a cripple. Small wonder that many stroke victims rarely ventured out of the house.

There was therefore a disillusionment with the traditional methods of stroke rehabilitation which had approached the problem in an arbitrary fashion. Gradually schools of thought developed which based treatment on the application of neurophysiological principles. Temple Fay, a neurosurgeon, studied primitive reflex patterns in animals and his observations led to the formulation of rehabilitative programmes which aimed to improve muscle tone and co-ordination of movement.[10] Brunnstrom[11] has made a detailed study of postural reflexes which occur in many hemiplegic patients. She utilises these associated reactions to encourage movement in the affected limbs. As voluntary movement is established, attempts are made to inhibit any spasticity which has developed.

Bertha Bobath and her husband have developed an approach to the hemiplegic patient which has attracted a lot of interest.[12] Her emphasis is on the development and control of normal patterns of movement as opposed to muscle strengthening. Because increased tone produces abnormal postural patterns, attempts are made to avoid spasticity by correct positioning of the patient in the early stages. The patient is positioned in bed with the arm extended, elevated and abducted; the trunk is extended, the hip held forwards and the knee slightly flexed. By preventing the development of an abnormal posture, it is hoped to avoid contractures, spasticity and bedsores. Activities which are said to increase spasticity are discouraged: no sandbags, as these will increase the likelihood of a plantar flexed foot, no oranges or rubber balls to squeeze as these are said to promote a spastic clenched fist. Doctors are tactfully asked not to encourage the patient to squeeze the good hand: squeezing has little prognostic value as the ability to let go is more important in useful manipulative function, and the patient may be tempted to go on squeezing the hand, with resultant unwanted hypertonicity.

As motor activity is dependent on sensory input, stimulation of the affected side is an important part of Bobath physiotherapy. Increased awareness of the affected side is achieved by encouraging the patient to look at the hemiplegic limbs (in order to reinforce the notion of 'self'); by doing exercises across the midline; by stimulation of the weak side and by encouraging bilateral activity. Other principles of treatment are the restoration of righting reactions, and balance reactions; the restriction of excessive activity of the good side, which the patient tends to use in preference to the weak side; and the initiation of limb movements starting with proximal muscle groups – the shoulder and hip girdles.

The aim of this type of physiotherapy is to achieve a more normal pattern of movement. The techniques would appear to be effective: there now seem to be fewer patients who develop a spastic gait. However, Bobath therapy has not yet been universally accepted. One criticism is that in the early stages of treatment independent mobility and personal independence are delayed, as the physiotherapist ensures that the patient has good postural balance before allowing him to stand and walk. This may not please the doctor, who may want to admit an acutely ill patient to that bed. And it may not please the patient, whose motivation to improve may diminish as he apparently makes little early progress. For hospitalised stroke patients who have not achieved independent mobility, the weekends are often interminably bleak; two days or more are spent without therapy, and the patient has to rely on others whenever he wants to be taken to the toilet, bathroom or dayroom. It is small wonder that his morale sags.

As yet we have no objective measures of the effectiveness of Bobath physiotherapy. The claim that it prevents, diminishes or abolishes spasticity could be measured objectively by devices which directly measure spasticity. The end results of treatment must also be assessed: are patients who have been treated by this method less likely to fall? Do they sustain fewer hip fractures? Does the apparent diminution in spasticity persist, or does therapy merely delay the development of the spastic pattern? Is the concentration on proximal muscle groups prior to distal ones a good thing, or would more patients develop useful hand function if manipulative activity was encouraged early? And are Bobath-treated patients more likely to return to social activities than those treated by other techniques or untreated stroke patients?

At present we have no facts to help us decide which type of physical therapy to administer. Much research is needed to answer other basic questions. Which patients should we treat and for how long? It seems that the amount of physiotherapy bears no relation to the patients' capacity for recovery; it is those with the greatest disability who receive most therapy.[13] We cannot yet identify accurately the patients who have good rehabilitative prospects. Simple, well validated prognostic indices of rehabilitation potential are urgently needed. We do not know whether hospital-based therapy is superior to domiciliary physiotherapy. In our experience, the rigours of an ambulance journey seem to be an important factor in producing spasticity: the therapist may spend a whole morning loosening up the patient, who then stiffens up again on the ambulance journey home. Add to this the high cost of bringing patients to hospital, and the case for initiating studies of home physiotherapy is overwhelming.

The assessment of physiotherapy is not easy. For scientific purity, untreated control groups are needed. However, few family doctors will be willing to subject elderly patients to an ambulance journey in order to attend a stroke rehabilitation centre where they may receive no active therapy. Moreover, physiotherapists will find it very difficult to leave people untreated, as they have seen too many patients who have developed avoidable complications which delay long-term recovery. We will therefore have to concentrate on assessing specific aspects of therapy and judging the success of treatment by measurable clinical end-points which relate to the practical daily activities of the patient.

At present the only certainty about physiotherapy is the extent of our ignorance. But there is currently an upsurge of interest in the evaluation of therapeutic techniques and many of the studies currently being done by physiotherapists themselves should yield interesting results.

## The Occupational Therapist

Occupational therapy began in TB sanatoria and long-stay wards with the introduction of craft work to relieve the patients' boredom and helplessness. The role of the occupational therapist has enlarged considerably over the years, but the concept of OTs as basket-makers who provide diversional therapy has been tenacious. In order to correct this widespread belief, let us examine how occupational therapists try to help our stroke patients.

Occupational therapists have three main roles: assessing patients and providing diagnostic help; improving the patient's ability to function; and preparing him and the family for going home. The basic thinking behind occupational therapy is that people treasure their independence: few people wish to be fed, washed and taken to the lavatory. Therefore, attempts are made to identify barriers to recovery, and to restore, encourage and maintain independence. This is achieved by helping the patient to re-learn everyday activities, providing aids and adaptions to help with mobility, and giving moral support.

Assessment mainly involves an analysis of how well a patient can perform daily living activities such as washing, dressing, cooking, going to the toilet. If a hemiplegic patient is unable to perform these tasks, it may be because of paralysis, but there are many other disabilities which are commonly overlooked. Parietal lobe disorder can cause perceptual problems and difficulties in performing purposeful movements in the absence of impaired sensation, motor power, co-ordination or comprehension (apraxia). These perceptual and praxic disorders are often poorly understood and misinterpreted. A dysphasic patient may be labelled demented not only because of his difficulty in understanding what is said and in formulating and vocalising a reply, but also because he cannot do simple tasks such as fastening a button – even though there is little or no motor weakness. By simple tests, the occupational therapist can diagnose the different kinds of apraxia, and inform the patient and staff that the disability has an organic basis. Other parietal disorders are misconstrued: patients with non-dominant hemisphere lesions may be thought to be 'poorly motivated' when in fact they may not be aware of the existence of their left side, because the mental image of self (the body schema) has been damaged. Others deny that they have had a stroke, or minimise its severity; these anosognostic phenomena may cause the patient to set unrealistic goals for himself or prevent him learning from his mistakes. Patients who are apparently incontinent may have spatial as well as praxic problems, and their 'incontinence' results from an inability to pick up a bottle or unfasten their buttons.

Before asking an occupational therapist to assess a patient's parietal function, the doctor must ensure that the patient is not deaf, demented or dysphasic: junior therapists may waste hours fruitlessly trying to assess these patients. It is sobering to realise that although we have known about parietal lobe disorders for decades, we still have no information on their incidence in a stroke population; whether perceptual, spatial and praxic problems improve with or without therapy; or how accurate are the various diagnostic tests for these under-diagnosed problems. Few doctors document parietal defects in the case notes: the neurological examination tends to be performed as if the cerebral cortex had not evolved!

Having established the nature of the impairment and the degree of functional disability, the therapist assesses the capacity for improvement and tries to help the patient overcome his handicap. The patient is encouraged to perform activities independently, and use is made of appropriate aids and gadgets.

Prior to discharge, the OT will do a home visit, usually with the patient, social worker and perhaps the physiotherapist. The need for installing aids is determined and any adaptions discussed. A downstairs lavatory may be needed; ramps can be fitted if steps to the front doors present difficulties; if the patient has to lead a wheelchair existence, doors may have to be widened. These home modifications are supplied by local authority social services in the United Kingdom and the hospital OT will work closely with the domiciliary OT who organises the provision of home aids. Much work is needed to determine which aids are most suitable for patients. Are the aids and adaptations actually used? Do they improve a patient's independence? Are they provided to those in greatest need? There are few published data on these and other aspects of the work of the occupational therapist. As yet we have no information on how much of an occupational therapist's effectiveness is due to her personality, and how much to the application of techniques or the provision of aids. Only by obtaining this information will the 'basket-maker' tag finally be removed.

### The Speech Therapist

The speech therapist is not usually actively involved in the multidisciplinary case conference in a geriatric unit. This is regrettable, as many stroke patients have language disorders and other problems, such as difficulty in swallowing, which the speech therapist may be able to ameliorate. She also has an important role in teaching the other staff how to communicate with the patient and in teaching the family what they can do to stimulate speech.

Is speech therapy effective? The first documented account of speech therapy appeared in the *American Journal of Insanity* in 1851,[14] when a 35-year-old blacksmith with valvular heart disease had a dysphasic stroke. His physician suggested writing and speaking exercises. Over a period of months, the patient's speech became increasingly fluent. Gradually methods of speech training became more complex and currently highly trained speech therapists may spend many hours assessing patients and attempting to improve language function. In the current climate of more critical evaluation of the role of the various profesional groups, the speech therapists have been the most closely scrutinised.

The present state of knowledge can be briefly summarised. Most dysphasic stroke patients improve during a course of speech therapy, and may improve sufficiently to speak intelligibly at home. Some patients make no significant recovery despite prolonged therapy. Others make a good recovery without any formal speech therapy. As recovery therefore cannot be attributed solely to rehabilitation, there has been some doubt cast on the effectiveness of speech therapy. However, a recent large-scale study from Italy[15] has shown that therapy given for 45-50 minutes three times a week, for over six months, resulted in restoration of speech that could be used in normal communication, and that this improvement was highly significantly better than that achieved in untreated control patients. Unfortunately, the two groups were not randomly allocated and the average age was only 50. None the less, until more persuasive data are forthcoming (and this will take many years), we can assume that formal speech therapy does work.

We do not know the optimum 'dose' of therapy – how long should each session last? How many sessions per week? How long should treatment continue? There are indications that the type of therapy given bears little relation to the aspect of speech which improves – for example, a therapist may concentrate on exercises to improve an aspect of comprehension, but the only measurable improvement may be in expression. This raises the question: is the therapy itself important or is it merely the stimulus to talk, and if so, could this be provided as effectively by an untrained but well motivated volunteer? A trial comparing outcome after speech therapy compared with volunteer therapy involved small numbers of patients who did not have comparable speech disorders.[16] Despite these and other shortcomings,the study has shown that volunteers appear to be as effective as professionals. Moreover, improvement can be shown even if many years have elapsed between the stroke and the initiation of amateur or professional therapy.[17]

Much more work is required to confirm these initial findings. Whilst we await the results of further studies, we should not neglect the basic aspects of caring for dysphasic patients. All too often these unfortunate people are ignored, or treated like children, or assumed to be mentally deficient, or shouted at because it is mistakenly believed that they are deaf. The speech therapist and the doctor have much work to do in educating all those who come into contact with the dysphasic stroke victim. The increasing number of volunteer 'speech after stroke' clubs[18] illustrate the need for volunteer and self-help groups. Speech therapists too are setting up social clubs for dysphasic patients who no longer receive formal therapy, and spouse groups where the practicalities of dysphasic care can be discussed.

The frustration experienced by a dysphasic stroke patient can be immense. The recent upsurge of interest in the best ways of helping these people is heartening.

## The Nurse

The nurse spends more time with the hospitalised patient and the family than any other person and the district nurse is often the only regular visitor to the stroke patient's home. Yet very little has been written about the nurse's role in rehabilitation and there have been strikingly few surveys of nursing skills and their relationship to the quality of the patient's life.

In the early stages of the stroke, the nurse has a vital role in preventing complications such as pressure sores, painful shoulders and contractures. Her observations are important in alerting the doctor to the onset of treatable but potentially fatal diseases such as chest infection and pulmonary embolus. In the elderly patients, pneumonia may develop with few of the textbook symptoms and signs. A rapid respiratory rate is a valuable sign and the importance of meticulous charting of respiration cannot be over-emphasised: pneumonia is one of the commonest causes of death in stroke patients who have survived the first days. As stroke patients may be unable to hold a thermometer under the tongue, axillary temperature recordings are often taken. The axillary temperature is usually lower on the affected side, and readings should always be taken from the sound side.[19]

Good nursing of stroke patients requires imagination and common sense. The nurse must ensure that dentures, hearing aids and spectacles are brought into hospital as early as possible. The patient's own shoes should be provided before the patient begins to walk; trying to walk in slippers does not make for a successful gait. Those few patients who are mobile but who require catheterisation should be provided with discreet catheter bags.

The siting of patients in the ward is particularly important. Patients with homonymous hemianopia or unilateral visual inattention should not be placed at the end of a ward where their only view is of a blank wall. In the first few days, lockers should be placed on the patient's good side, where he can see a drink and reach for it. Far too many patients become dehydrated in the first week of a stroke. The locker should be put back on the hemiplegic side after the early stages, to reinforce bilaterality and to encourage the patient to move across the midline to his weak side.

The nurse new to rehabilitation learns a different approach to the elderly patient. Previously she will have been taught to do everything for him, now she has to learn progressive disengagement, of encouraging the patient to do things independently. This can be difficult: patients and their families expect nurses to do things for them, and many patients who are capable of doing everyday activities for the occupational therapist will wait for the nurse to help them perform these tasks. The practicalities of geriatric care sometimes militate against successful nursing. If a ward is inadequately staffed, the nurse will be tempted to take patients to the toilet or day-room in a wheelchair rather than encourage them to walk; to dress and fasten buttons for them; and not to take the time and patience needed to encourage dysphasic patients to communicate.

The nurse has an important role in educating the family: she can clear up misunderstandings about aphasia, agnosia and apraxia and many other perplexing features of cerebrovascular disease. She should increasingly involve the family in practical patient care. Before the patient is discharged, the nurse should ensure that he has had trial days and week-ends at home, and discuss with the family any problems that may have arisen during these periods. The transition from hospital to home life is a time of considerable anxiety to stroke families and everything possible should be done to ease their worries.

Several surveys have shown that about half of all stroke patients are not admitted acutely to hospital, and that admission is influenced more by social than medical considerations. Many hospital patients will have some disability on discharge. With the increasing trend towards earlier discharge and 'hospitals at home' it is clear that the district nurse and the health visitor will have a large and increasingly important role in stroke care. Little is known about the effectiveness of district nurses in managing stroke patients. One community study of 30 stroke patients, the majority of whom were over 65 years of age, showed that most of the district nurses involved in care were trained twenty years ago.[20] Many of them were not familiar with new developments in techniques of stroke rehabilitation. The general practitioners involved had only a vague idea about the role of the district nurse in looking after stroke patients. Ideally, the good district nurse should be familiar with the practical aspects of physiotherapy, occupational therapy, speech therapy and psychological support. There is much room for further development of domiciliary rehabilitation of stroke.

## The Social Worker

The first controlled study of social work in the elderly which was conducted in this country showed that highly trained social workers were more effective than untrained local authority workers in meeting the needs of old people.[21] However, this may have been due to the differences in size of case-loads in the two groups.[22] As with other members of the therapeutic team, there has been much assertion but little documentation of the role or effectiveness of social workers in dealing with stroke patients.

In one social work journal, there was only one article devoted to stroke in an 18-year period,[23] yet stroke is the major cause of serious physical disability in our community. The few articles which have been published tend to concentrate on the emotional aspects of stroke illness; there is far less written on the practical help which social workers can provide. So what do social workers actually do?

There are three components of social work: assessment, emotional support and practical support. In order to compile her report, the social worker collects information from the patient, the family, other sources outside hospital and from the various members of the rehabilitation team. By piecing together this data, she is able to appraise the overall situation and to make recommendations which will help the doctor to decide how to plan not only the patient's discharge (which is usually relatively easy) but also the more difficult task of after-care. There are certain basic facts that the doctor must know: Who is at home with the patient? Is the bed upstairs or downstairs? Is there a downstairs toilet? A social network diagram has been recommended as a succinct way of tabulating the relevant social details.[24]

The impact of stroke can be as great on the family as on the stricken individual. Families know very little about the physical aspects of stroke, and much less about the normal emotional reactions to stroke. By an understanding of these psychological aspects, the social worker may be able to help the family come to terms with the illness and prepare it for the adjustments needed when the patient comes home.

Both patients and their families undergo a grief reaction after a stroke. This usually follows a predictable pattern, although the time scale for the development of the different features may vary from person to person. After the initial shock, there is relief that the person has survived. There follows a period of concern about the eventual outcome, and then a phase of disbelief and anger. The anger may be directed towards the doctors, nurses and therapists who must be aware of this reaction as normal so that they do not take offence and in order that they may sympathise with and offer help to the relatives. Later there is realisation that the patient will probably be permanently disabled; awareness of the implications that this has for their life-style; and doubts about their own capacity to cope. Over a long period, then, the family may need emotional support. In hospital, all the staff who come into contact with the family will provide this support: it is not the exclusive responsibility of the social worker. Whether more effective support is provided by fully trained than by untrained workers is open to question. We do not know if the counselling of a professional improves the social activities of patient or family. Nor do we have much information on the attitude of elderly patients and relatives to social workers. It may be that tangible benefits (such as the installation of a telephone or the organisation of holiday care) may be more appreciated than visits aimed at providing psychological support. A recent development is the increasing numbers of spouse groups, where relatives can get things off their chest and discuss matters of mutual interest. In some areas, social workers organise these; in others they are arranged by the non-professionals who run stroke clubs.

On the practical side the social worker can contribute towards arranging as early a discharge as is practicable and can arrange for residential home accommodation for those patients who cannot cope alone at home. If a person is able to go home, the social workers liaises with social services to provide outside help such as home helps, meals on wheels, luncheon clubs and attendance at day centres. She can also arrange for relief or holiday admission of those patients who do not need medical, nursing or physical therapy to local authority homes, in order that relatives can have a regular break. She also has an important role in ensuring that relatives get all the allowances to which they are entitled, and in providing aids and adaptations. When she eventually closes the case, she may arrange for continuing care by volunteer organisations.

This is the theory: how much practical help is actually provided will depend on the ability and enthusiasm of the individual social workers and on the financial position of the local authority. The effectiveness of the provision of aid is unknown. Articulate accounts of the difficulties, delays and confusion encountered by relatives in obtaining such simple items as an orthopaedic chair suggest that there is no room for complacency.[25] The whole area of social and psychological support for stricken families needs to be examined carefully.

## The Doctor and the Patient

One of the many attractive features of geriatric medicine is that it enables the physician to practice 'whole person' medicine. What does this actually mean with regard to the stroke patient? So far we have critically discussed the various members of the rehabilitation team and their roles: the physiotherapist who aims to improve balance and control of movement; the occupational therapist who assesses perceptual disorders and the performance of daily living activities and prepares the patient for going home; the speech therapist who tries to improve the patient's use of language; the social worker who helps with the emotional and practical aspects of stroke; and the nurse who, in addition to her technical skills, is so important in providing the *ambiance* in which the stroke patient can recover to his full capacity. As we have seen, the doctor has little in the way of drug therapy to help the stroke vicitm, although there may be scope for secondary prevention. His main functions are in providing explanation, reassurance and sensible advice and ensuring that the patient and family are well supported by the various statutory and voluntary agencies.

Here we are concerned more with the art of medicine than with the science: 'A body yet distemper'd which to his former strength may be restored with good advice and little medicine'.[26]

To provide effective advice and reassurance, the doctor must be familiar with the anxieties of the stroke patient and family. This is best ascertained by simply asking, 'What is the thing that troubles you most?' This often provides surprising answers: 'loneliness', 'money' and 'drooling from my mouth' often crop up when one might expect 'a useless arm' to be the main problem. Unfortunately, many patients do not mention their real worries: they may be too anxious; they may think that the problems are too trivial to tell the doctor, they may perceive a social distance between themselves and the doctor or may not express themselves in words that the doctor understands. The doctor can often be helped by nurses, therapists and social workers with whom patients may find communication easier.

Many novelists and playwrights have used stroke victims as characters – for example, Kingsley Amis's novel *Ending Up*[27] can teach us much more about dysphasia than many a neurological text. Books and articles written by stroke patients themselves are often most instructive. Anthony Richardson[28] vividly describes the problems of stroke and his determination to overcome them:

> I intend, with God's grace, to return to a normal life. I may stagger and lurch and stutter. I may dribble out of the corner of my mouth and find myself blundering into my neighbour. I may go up and down stairs like a crab and hobble about like a marionette, but I'm not going to adopt the pose of an invalid. I just won't have it.

Typical questions asked by stroke patients include: What has happened? Why? Why has it happened to me? Will it happen again, and if so, will it kill me? Am I going to get better? How long will it take? How will I adjust to my disability?

There is much ignorance concerning the nature and causes of stroke. Many people confuse stroke with myocardial infarction, or indeed with any type of thrombosis, be it arterial or venous. The doctor should explain in simple terms the mechanism of haemorrhagic and occlusive stroke. Jargon is to be avoided as even common medical words are often poorly understood by the layman. Hypertension may be interpreted as meaning resulting from stress or tension. There is a common belief, reinforced by the news media, that tension, overwork or a traumatic event can precipitate a stroke. There is no good evidence to support this. In a study of 300 patients, a clear temporal correlation betwen a disturbing event and the occurrence of stroke was found in less than 1 per cent.[29] The belief that stress causes stroke is so deep-seated that many stroke patients impose unnecessary restrictions on their activity – indeed, the self-imposed limitations may exceed those caused by the physical disability. Further limitations are imposed by well-meaning members of the family, and even by doctors, whose advice to 'take it easy' may condemn a person to a grey existence as a virtual prisoner in his own home.

Once over the initial shock of the stroke the patient and family often ask themselves what they have done to deserve being struck down. Many see strokes as a form of punishment for real or imagined sins of omission or commission. One man looked in the mirror shortly after his stroke and said to himself: 'It serves you right, you rotten bastard, for all your lack of love and understanding.'[28] The doctor's reassurance that stroke is not a form of retribution may ease guilt and self-recrimination. Activities believed to cause stroke are often studiously avoided by patients wishing to avoid further strokes. There is a common belief that as stroke is caused by something snapping at the back of the head, bending the head may cause further strokes. The dizziness caused by vertebrobasilar insufficiency that is so common in the elderly reinforces this fear. Consequently the person avoids bending whenever possible: dropped items remain on the floor; gardens are untended; shoe-laces are tied by others, reinforcing the feeling of dependence and reducing further the patient's self-esteem. It is also worth asking people what they were doing at the time of the stroke, as many assume that this activity caused the attack. One patient I met was never enthusiastic about salad. His wife eventually persuaded him into eating some lettuce, and he sustained a stroke shortly afterwards. He could never be persuaded to eat lettuce again, and the wife was convinced that her nagging had effected the stroke. It is hard to help people whose stroke occurred during coitus to resume an active sex life.

Having recovered from a stroke, a major worry is whether and when a further stroke will occur. This is particularly so in those who have had two strokes. There is a widespread belief that the third stroke is always fatal, and explaining that a third stroke may never occur, and that some people have many little strokes may go some way towards alleviating the patient's anxiety. People are also naturally concerned about the speed and degree of recovery. Many believe that as the stroke came on suddenly, recovery will be just as dramatic and they look forward to that morning when the bad nightmare is over and they will wake up completely cured. It must be constantly emphasised that recovery is almost invariably gradual, and that it may continue for many months or years. The patient must be prepared for the likely pattern and extent of recovery: most will be able to walk again, but useful hand function is uncommon and should be considered a bonus. None the less, hand exercises should be diligently adhered to in order to prevent regression of mobility. There are several causes of embarrassment, anxiety and depression with which the physician must be familiar. Emotional lability is common, and the tendency to cry or sometimes to laugh inappropriately worries many patients and their relatives. It may be feared that this is a sign of impending madness, and explanation that it is as much a feature of stroke as is the weak arm and that it will improve with time will take a lot of the emotional heat out of this distresssing complaint. Depression is almost universal, though perhaps less marked in the more philosophical elderly person than in the younger stroke victim, and may require drug therapy. Unilateral facial weakness horrifies some patients. Whereas the hospital doctor may be interested in the differences between an upper and a lower motor neurone seventh nerve weakness, the patient finds facial asymmetry embarrassing and may wonder why no one does anything about it. Applying ice to the weak part of the face and then brushing it does seem to improve the muscle tone, but how much of this recovery is spontaneous has not been assessed. Problems with communication cause enormous frustration to patient and family, and friends who may think the patient has become insane or who are not emotionally equipped to cope with dysphasia, often stop visiting.

The hemiplegic arm is a major preoccupation. Complete recovery is rare; what improvement does occur is slow, and mainly involves proximal muscle groups. This pattern of recovery must be constantly emphasised, as must a more hopeful viewpoint. Even if the manipulative function is poor, the hand can be often used to anchor things. If the arm remains totally useless, independence can be achieved by the provision of the many aids and appliances which are available.

Although some leg use usually recovers, a poor gait pattern may cause embarrassment and therefore prevent the patient from going out.

A major fear is of falling ('the abiding menace, to be circumvented at all costs. At the least it can mean loss of confidence, at the most serious injury.').[28] The family doctor must be alert to factors in the house which may make the patient slip or trip, and the carer must be familiar with the technique of lifting stroke patients.

In addition to providing explanation and reassurance, the doctor can help in other ways. He can ensure that the family has explanatory booklets which give practical advice on the physical, psychological and social difficulties produced by stroke.[30] He can introduce the patient and family to the various clubs that offer help – stroke clubs, volunteer speech groups, groups for relatives. He can arrange for continuing medical care at day hospitals, and social support at day centres. He can organise home visits by volunteers.

## Conclusion

Stroke rehabilitation is a rapidly developing area of medicine. There is much that we do not know, and it may be that some of our present practices will be discarded in the future. We still do not know how much successful rehabilitation is effected by the interest, enthusiasm and compassion of the rehabilitation team, and how much (if any) is a result of applying specialised techniques. Much work needs to be done, but even at this early stage it appears justified to allow a faint glimmer of excitement to penetrate the curtain of caution.

## References

1. Mushet, W.B. (1864) *A Practical Treatise on Apoplexy*, John Churchill & Sons, London
2. Thomas, D.J. Marshall, J., Ross Russell, R.W., Wetherley-Mein, G., Du Boulay, G.H. Pearson, T.C., Symon, L., and Zilkha, G. (1977) 'Effect of Haematocrit on Cerebral Blood-flow in Man', *Lancet, ii*, 941-3
3. Poe, W.D. (1972) 'Marantology, a Needed Speciality', *New England Journal of Medicine, 286*, 102-3
4. Gowers, W.R. (1888) *A Manual of Diseases of the Nervous System*, Churchill, London
5. Westcott, E.J. (1967) 'Traditional Exercise Regimens for the Hemiplegic Patient', *American Journal of Physical Medicine, 46*, 1012-23
6. Coulter, J.S. (1939) in *Principles and Practice of Physical Therapy*, W.F. Prior, Maryland, vol. 3, pp. 46-50
7. Drinken, H. (1947) 'The Evaluation of Disability and Treatment in Hemiplegia', *Archives of Physical Medicine, 28,* 263-72
8. Hodkinson, H.M., and Brain, A.T. (1967) 'Unilateral Osteoporosis in Long-

standing Hemiplegia in the Elderly', *Journal of the American Geriatric Society, 15*, 59-64
9. Mulley G.P., and Espley, A. (1979) 'Hip Fracture after Hemiplegia', *Postgraduate Medical Journal, 55*, 264-5
10. Page, D. (1967) 'Neuromuscular Reflex Therapy as an Approach to Patient Care', *American Journal of Physical Medicine, 46*, 816-21
11. Brunnstrom, S. (1956) 'Associated Reactions of the Upper Extremity in Adult Patients with Hemiplegia: an Approach to Training', *Physical Therapy Review, 36*, 225-36
12. Bobath, B. (1978) *Adult Hemiplegia: Evaluation and Treatment*, 2nd edn, Heinemann, London
13. Brocklehurst, J.C. Andrews, K., Richards, B., Laycock, P.J. (1978) 'How Much Physical Therapy for Patients with Stroke?' *British Medical Journal, 1*, 1307-10
14. Hun, T. (1851) 'A Case of Amnesia', *American Journal of Insanity, 7*, 358-63
15. Basso, A., Capitani, E., Vignolo, L.A. (1979) 'Influence of Rehabilitation on Language Skills in Aphasic Patients. A Controlled Study', *Archives of Neurology, 36*, 190-6
16. Meikle, M., Wechsler, E., Tupper, A., Benenson, M., Butler, J., Mulhall, D., and Stern, G. (1978) 'Comparative Trial of Volunteer and Professional Treatments of Dysphasia after Stroke', *British Medical Journal, 2*, 87-9
17. David, R.M., Enderby. P., Bainton, D. (1979) 'Progress Report on an Evaluation of Speech Therapy for Dysphasia', *British Journal of Disorders of Communication, 14*, 85-8
18. Griffith, V.E. (1975) 'Volunteer Scheme for Dysphasia and Allied Problems in Stroke Patients', *British Medical Journal, 3*, 633-5
19. Mulley, G.P. (1980) 'Axillary Temperature Differences in Hemiplegia', *Postgraduate Medical Journal, 56*, 248-9
20. Kratz, C.R. (1978) *Care of the Long-term Sick in the Community*, Churchill Livingstone, Edinburgh
21. Goldberg, E.M., Mortimer, A., Williams, B.T. (1970) *Helping the Aged. A Field Experiment in Social Work*, National Institute of Social Work Library No. 19 Allen and Unwin, London
22. Cochrane, A.L.(1972) *Effectiveness and Efficiency. Random Reflections on Health Services*, The Nuffield Provincial Hospitals Trust
23. Hartshorn, A. (1967) 'The Role of the Social Worker in the Treatment of Stroke Illness', *Medical Social Work, 20*, 3-12
24. Capildeo, R., Court, C., Rose, C.F. (1976) 'Social Network Diagram', *British Medical Journal, 1*, 143-4
25. Wicke, M. (1978) 'Time to Go Home', *New Age* (Summer), 20-1
26. Shakespeare, W. *Henry IV*, Part 2
27. Amis, K. (1974) *Ending Up*, Cape, London
28. Richardson, A. (1959) *Never Say Die. A Return to Everyday Living for the Partly Disabled*, Max Parrish, London
29. Ullman, M. (1962) *Behavioural Changes in Patients Following Strokes*, C.C. Thomas, Springfield, Illinois
30. Mulley, G.P. (1978) *Stroke. A Handbook for the Patient's Family*, Chest, Heart and Stroke Association, London

# 3 THE ELDERLY IN A COLD ENVIRONMENT

A.N. Exton-Smith

A well known characteristic of ageing is the impairment in physiological systems which leads to a diminished control of homeostasis. Thus all functions in the nervous system show a progressive decline throughout adult life. These insidious and progressive changes are reflected by a steady decline in the adaptability of the individual and by a parallel increase in susceptibility to environmental stress. Homeostasis is still maintained, but with increasing difficulty as the years pass, since there is a slow erosion of the capacity for mental and physical adaptation to the strains imposed by the external environment.

The ecological relationships with which we are concerned is the effect of a cold environment on the maintenance of the internal temperature of the body. The healthy young adult can withstand exposure to severe degrees of cold stress and make the necessary physiological adjustments which maintain his 'core' or deep body temperature. In the elderly even minor degrees of cold exposure can lead to a fall in deep body temperature; the condition of accidental hypothermia exists when the core temperature drops below the arbitrarily defined limit of 35.0°C. The term accidental hypothermia is used to indicate that the lowering of body temperature is unintentional and it is to be distinguished from hypothermia which is induced therapeutically. It became recognised in the United Kingdom in the early 1960s as a problem particularly affecting old people.

## Temperature Regulation

### *Normal Regulation of Body Temperature*

The capacity to maintain a stable deep body temperature or homeothermy is an evolutionary development found only in birds and other mammals. Ideally in these animals all body tissues would be maintained at optimum temperature, but this would be costly in energy production and it would also be difficult to achieve. Thus in man and other homeothermic animals the deep body or core temperature is controlled and the superficial or body shell is used as a variable insulator. The heart and circulation act as a heat exchange system.

The tissues situated in the outer shell of the body consist of the skin, subcutaneous tissue and superficial layers of muscle. Those in the core of the body include the brain, heart, liver, kidneys, pancreas and the gastrointestinal tract. It is the vital core of the body which is maintained at a temperature of 37.0°C or close to this level. Body temperature is usually measured by placing a mercury-in-glass clinical thermometer in the mouth, but this temperature may be affected by hot or cold food and drinks and by previous mouth breathing. The use of a clinical thermometer placed in the rectum is a more reliable indicator of the deep body temperature. The temperature of freshly voided urine also provides a reliable measure. It is within about 0.1°C of the rectal temperature.[1] When a normal young adult is exposed to cold for a period of 1½ to 2 hours the mouth temperature may fall below 35.0°C but this individual is not hypothermic since the rectal or urine temperature is still maintained at 37.°C. There is a temperature difference between the deep tissues and the surface of the body and heat flows down a gradient to the skin and hence by convection and radiation from the surface of the body. In a state of thermal comfort the skin temperature is approximately 33°C and the core skin temperature gradient is about 4°C.[2] In a warm environment the blood flow through the skin is increased to promote the transfer of heat to the body surface; conversely, under cool conditions the blood flow is reduced to conserve heat. This vasomotor regulation is capable of maintaining homeothermy over a fairly wide range of environmental temperatures. Under conditions of extremely high or low external temperatures protection against hyperthermia and hypothermia is achieved by the operation of the additional mechanisms of sweating and shivering. In civilised societies man is able to live almost entirely within the vasomotor control zone without the operation of these emergency mechanisms by adapting his immediate environment through appropriate clothing, heating and air conditioning.

The maintenance of a relatively constant deep body temperature of 37°C depends upon the balance of heat gain and heat loss from the whole body. This balance is under the control of the nervous system and in particular of the hypothalamus, which is the main thermoregulatory centre of the brain. The input to the hypothalamic controller comes from the thermo-sensitive end organs in the skin and from the thermo-sensors mainly within the hypothalamus, particularly in the anterior region. The output from the hypothalamus is mediated through the autonomic effector system controlling peripheral blood flow, pilo-erection and sweating and through actions on the endocrine glands and voluntary muscles influencing heat production. In man, vasomotor control in the skin depends on vasoconstrictor autonomic nerves and on a vasodilator mechanism. The vasoconstrictor mechanism predominates in the hands and the feet and is only weakly represented in the proximal parts and the trunk.

In a person who feels cold but who is not shivering blood flow in the hands is approximately 1ml/100ml hand tissue/min. Under thermally neutral conditions it is usually in the range of 4-10 ml and when the body is heated it rises to over 40 ml.[3] The stimulus to vasoconstriction arises mainly from the cold receptors in the skin. Within the vasomotor control zone hand blood flow is very sensitive to small changes in skin temperature in the rest of the body, marked vasoconstriction and vasodilation being elicited by minor degrees of cooling and warming respectively.

Metabolic heat production can be increased voluntarily by exercise or involuntarily by a cold environment using increased activity in skeletal muscle culminating in shivering. This specialised form of muscular activity is mediated through somatic, not autonomic, nerves. It consists of an uncoordinated pattern in which groups of muscle fibres within a muscle contract and relax out of phase with each other. The effect of this increased muscular activity is increased heat production which for periods of a few minutes may amount to five times the resting metabolic rate.[2] Characteristically shivering occurs in bursts and it cannot be sustained a maximum level for long, so the overall heat production due to shivering may amount to three times the resting level when measured over a period of one hour. It is evoked by activity of the cold receptors in the skin and probably by a fall in central temperature in the hypothalamic region. At a core body temperature below about 32°C the shivering action is abolished and thermogenesis then depends on increased skeletal muscle tone. Long-term exposure to cold leads to increased output of thyroxine and the catecholamines, adrenalin and noradrenalin.

### *Impairment of Thermoregulatory Function*

An early observation of the effect of cold exposure on body temperature in old people showed that they suffered from impairment of temperature homeostasis.[4] Thirteen aged subjects (57-91 years old) were exposed to an ambient temperature of -15° to -9°C for 45-120 minutes and the physiological responses were compared with those of young adults (22-36 years) similarly exposed. Although the aged subjects experienced less discomfort than the young and they did not shiver, they were less able to maintain their deep body temperature. Similar observations were made by workers in Oxford in investigations of temperature regulation in the survivors of accidental hypothermia.[5] The resting deep body temperature of the survivors was low and on exposure to cold it fell progressively and abnormally. By contrast, elderly control subjects who had not experienced hypothermia showed responses similar to those of young healthy adults. Thus the defect in temperature regulation in the survivors of accidental hypothermia persists and these old people are probably at risk from another episode of hypothermia when exposed to only moderate cold. It is not clear, however, from these findings to what extent impaired homeostasis is a feature of ageing and whether it occurs in marked degree in people who are likely to develop hypothermia on cold exposure.

The development of the Uritemp technique by Dr Ronald Fox of the Medical Research Council provided a practical means of measuring deep body temperature in old people living at home.[6] The Nuffield Foundation supported the first large-scale domiciliary survey of environmental and body temperatures in old people during the first three months of 1972.[1] The body temperatures measured were those of the mouth, hand and urine and the environmental temperatures included those of the living-room, the bedroom and the outdoor temperature. Sets of temperature recordings were made both morning and evening. The national survey was based on 1,020 old people living in their own homes in centres throughout the British Isles, a further 1,000 old people living in the London Borough of Camden were investigated in the same period. The winter environmental temperatures in 1972 were slightly higher than average, but in 75 per cent of cases the living-room temperatures in the morning were at or below 18.3°C, the minimum recommended by the Parker Morris Report for Council Housing,[7] and in 10 per cent the room temperatures were very cold, at or below 12°C. Only 0.5 per cent of the subjects were hypothermic with a urine temperature of less than 35.0°C and all these subjects had temperatures within the range of 34.2 to 34.9°C. However, 10 per cent of the subjects both in the national study and in the Camden study had urine temperatures of between 35°C and 35.5°C. These subjects in the 'low' temperature group were thought to have some degree of thermoregulatory failure as shown by the inability to maintain an adequate core-periphery temperature gradient. The mean difference between the urine temperature and the hand temperature in the low-temperature group was 2.9°C, compared with 4.6°C for those in the normal temperature group in whom deep body temperatures were 36.0°C and above. Significant correlations with decreasing deep body temperature were advancing age, the hands feeling cold, preference for a warmer environment and the receipt of supplementary benefit. Urine and hand temperatures showed a negative correlation with age, but there was no significant relationship between mouth and room temperatures and advancing age. The absence of a relationship between room temperature and age seems to exclude one hypothesis for the decline of deep body temperature with age, namely, it is simply due to the older people living in colder accommodation. The salient feature of this study was the finding that only a small proportion of old people at home suffer from hypothermia. Large numbers of old people, however, are on the borderline of hypothermia with low deep body temperatures of less than 35.5°C. These people are at risk not only because they are less successful in conserving body heat, as shown by an inability to maintain an adequate core to shell temperature gradient, but also because they have a proportionally lower body heat content.

These studies of body and environmental temperatures of old people at home provided a naturally occurring physiological experiment in which it has been shown that there is often impairment of thermoregulatory capacity when the elderly are subject to mild or moderate degrees of cold stress. The nature of this physiological impairment was further investigated following the domiciliary survey when 150 of the Camden subjects agreed to attend the Geriatric Department at University College Hospital. Tests of thermoregulatory function were made by measuring physiological responses to a cycle of neutral, cool and warm environments created by a specially designed air-conditioned bed.[8] With the view to reducing stress to a minimum, attention was confined to the vasomotor zone of thermoregulation. Following a neutral phase during which the air temperature was maintained at 30°C, it was reduced to 15°C for a period of 16 minutes – which represents only a mild degree of cold stress since, as we have seen, some 40-50 per cent of people occupy rooms below this temperature in the winter. The air temperature was then raised to 45°C for 46 minutes or until the subject sweated, whichever occurred first. Vasomotor control was investigated by measuring the hand blood flow using a plethysmograph. The normal pattern of hand blood flow which is found in young subjects who were used for comparison consists of a reduction in flow on cooling and an elevation of blood flow on warming. Approximately half the elderly subjects, however, had an abnormal pattern of peripheral blood flow in which there was no reduction of flow on cooling (non-constrictor response). Moreover, there was evidence of other defects in thermoregulation in the old people: two-fifths of the men and three-fifths of the women failed to sweat on warming and the shivering reaction was absent in all but 12 per cent of the old people tested. The frequent absence of shivering in old people exposed to cold has been noted by other observers.[9] When the results of the thermoregulatory tests were related to the domiciliary temperature measurement it was found that there was evidence of autonomic dysfunction (non-constrictor peripheral blood flow patterns, failure to sweat on warming and the presence of postural hypotension) in all but one of the twelve subjects who had deep body temperatures below 35.5°C; this single subject had true hypothermia (urine temperature 34.4°C) and this was probably attributable to the fact that she was living in an extremely low room temperature. In contrast, evidence of autonomic dysfunction was much less frequently seen in subjects who had a normal deep body temperature.

Caution must be exercised in interpreting results of cross-sectional studies when comparison is made between old and young individuals. True age changes in physiological performances can only be determined accurately by longitudinal studies in which serial measurements are made on the same individual at two points of time.[10] An opportunity arose for studying on a longitudinal basis changes in thermoregulatory function when 43 of the Camden subjects were reinvestigated four years later using the same physiological techniques which were previously employed.[11] The domiciliary survey in the winter months of 1976 showed that the environmental and living-room temperatures and the oral, hand and urine temperatures were not significantly different from those recorded in 1972. Detailed analysis of the results of the thermoregulatory function tests however, showed that significant changes had occurred during the four-year period: in 1976 a significantly higher proportion of the old people had low resting peripheral blood flows (less than 5 ml/100 ml hand tissue/minute); a higher proportion had a non-constrictor response on cooling; the deep body temperature at sweat onset was significantly higher in 1976 than in 1972; a significantly higher proportion of the subjects in 1976 had postural hypotension with a fall in systolic blood pressure $>$ 20 mm Hg, and the weighted total body measurement of skin temperature obtained in the bed test showed that the core-peripheral temperature gradient was significantly smaller in 1976 during the resting, neutral and cooling stages.

Thus from the results of the physiological studies made on the Camden volunteers we have shown on a cross-sectional and longitudinal basis that there is an age-related decline in autonomic nervous function which leads to impairment of thermoregulatory capacity in a high proportion of old people.

### *Impairment of Thermal Perception*

In addition to the changes in autonomic function which lead to impairment of thermoregulatory capacity, many old people have a diminished sensitivity to cold. Tests of digital thermosensation show that young people can perceive mean temperature differences of about 0.8°C, whereas elderly subjects can discriminate only between mean temperatures of 2.1°C and some are unable to perceive differences of 5°C or more.[11] In a series of experiments on groups of young and elderly subjects exposed to a range of ambient temperatures of 12° – 24°C temperature discrimination by the elderly was always worse than for the younger subjects. Moreover, in both groups discrimination deteriorated markedly in the coldest ambient conditions.[12] It is likely that a lessened sensitivity to cold is one of the reasons why relatively large numbers of old people appear to be able to tolerate cold conditions without discomfort. Nevertheless, such individuals may be at risk of overtaxing the heat-conserving capacity of a failing thermoregulatory system.

## Hypothermia

A crucial issue which faces the epidemiologist is how to define a clinical case. Is it to be regarded as a dichotomy or as a continuum?[13] Are those individuals who comprise 0.5 per cent of the population and who have deep body temperatures below 35.0°C merely the tail end of a normal distribution as the national and Camden studies would suggest, or are they abnormal in some way?

There are four types of criteria on which the definition can be approached – statistical, clinical, prognostic and operational.[13] The nature of the criteria used depends upon the variable being studied, but none is entirely satisfactory. In clinical practice dichotomy is unavoidable and it is necessary to fix a limit beyond which a pathological condition is likely to be present and treatment of the individual may be required. In the case of epidemiological studies of arterial blood pressure, for example, the systolic pressure of 150 mm Hg in a man aged 50 is 'statistically' normal, but it is known that this individual has a greater risk of ischaemic heart disease than the man with the lower blood pressure. Thus if prognostic criteria are to be adopted for the definition of hypertension, follow-up studies are needed to determine the levels of blood pressure above which the risk of complications becomes unacceptable.

The definition of hypothermia as a deep body temperature below 35.0°C is similarly based on clinical and prognostic criteria. It is known that individuals with deep body temperatures below 35°C are more likely to have clinical manifestations, complications are more frequent and the mortality rates are higher than for those with normal body temperatures. Thus in the surveys of patients with hypothermia admitted to hospital carried out on behalf of the Royal College of Physicians[14,15] there was a close relationship between levels of rectal temperature and mortality. In the second survey[15] the mortality rate was 75 per cent for elderly patients with deep body temperatures on admission below 30°C and 39 per cent for those with temperatures of 30-34.9°C; these rates were significantly higher than for patients whose temperatures were 35-35.9°C (29.4 per cent) and above 36.0°C (27.5 per cent).

*Prevalence* Although domiciliary surveys indicate that hypothermia in the elderly population is comparatively rare, it is much more frequently seen in patients admitted to hospital. In the first Royal College of Physicians' Survey carried out in ten hospitals in England and Scotland during a three-month period in the winter of 1965 it was found that 126 patients of all ages were suffering from hypothermia; that is, the incidence was 0.68 per cent of all patients admitted. Forty-two per cent were over the age of 65 and the incidence in this age group was 1.2 per cent. Extrapolating to the country as a whole, it was calculated that about 3,800 elderly patients were admitted to hospital with hypothermia during the three months of the survey. The importance of low environmental temperature was established by comparing the number of hypothermic admissions per week with the mean minimal environmental temperature for all areas during that week. On the coldest week of the survey, with a mean minimal environmental temperature of -4.0°C, 19 hypothermic patients were admitted, the highest number for any one week. During the three weeks when the mean minimum temperature exceeded +4°C, hypothermic admissions averaged only 4 per week. It can be concluded from these observations that there is a clear relationship between the incidence of hypothermia and environmental temperature. Some cases of hypothermia, however, occurred in climatic conditions which were mild. It was also noted that although the majority of patients were admitted as emergencies, some patients had hypothermia when admitted from the waiting list.

Ten years later, in a second Royal College of Physicians study[15] conducted at University College Hospital and the Royal Free Hospital, London, measurements of rectal temperature in all patients over the age of 65 admitted in January to April 1975 showed that 3.6 per cent of patients had hypothermia, a prevalence considerably higher than that found in the previous study. Though deep body temperature was significantly correlated with cold exposure immediately preceding admission and with living alone, three-quarters of the patients suffering from cold exposure were exposed to cold indoors.

*Aetiology*. Two Royal College of Physicians studies[14, 15] and the reports of clinical cases of hypothermia,[16, 17, 18] show that exposure to cold is an overriding cause. A common story is of an old person who falls after attempting to get out of bed at night; he remains on the floor for several hours, often partly clad, and is discovered the next day by a relative, neighbour or home help. Important contributory factors increasing the risk of cold exposure in old people are physical conditions associated with falls (vertigo, visual defects, postural instability, orthostatic hypotension, arthritis and difficulty in getting about in the dark) and the cold conditions in which many old people live in winter.[1] For elderly people who sustain a fall at night the exposure is likely to be longer when the individual lives alone and is socially isolated. In other instances the cold exposure is less severe and hypothermia develops when the old person is in bed and apparently well covered with clothes. In these instances insufficient body heat is generated so that even good external insulation is ineffective.

When sufficiently severe, exposure to cold alone can lead to accidental hypothermia. This condition is sometimes known as primary hypothermia and it is diagnosed in the absence of any significant pathological condition which could account for the hypothermia. A diagnosis of primary hypothermia was made in 20 per cent of the patients of all ages reported in the first Royal College of Physicians survey and in 33 per cent of the elderly patients described in the second study. Even in these cases, however, when old people are the victims, it is likely that the age-related physiological impairment of thermoregulation and the diminished sensitivity to cold are important factors increasing the liability to hypothermia.

In the majority of cases of old people admitted to hospital suffering from accidental hypothermia, pathological conditions are present. These conditions are involve a number of bodily systems. In the endocrine disorders, myxoedema and hypopituitarism, hypothermia is the result of diminished metabolic heat production. In diabetes mellitus tests of autonomic function[19] show a high frequency of autonomic neuropathy which leads to impairment of thermoregulation. The impairment of thermoregulation is often overlooked in Wernicke's encephalopathy and hypothermia is not uncommon.[20] It is usually due to vitamin $B_1$ deficiency often associated with alcoholism and is characterised by petechial haemorrhages in the walls of the third ventricle, the hypothalamus and mammillary bodies. Patients with confusional states and dementia may be unaware of environmental hazards and do not adequately protect themselves against the cold. In addition there is some evidence for impairment of temperature regulation in dementia.[21] Psychotropic drugs, especially the phenothiazines, which are prescribed for these conditions may also effect thermoregulation. Bronchopneumonia may precipitate hypothermia and it usually develops insidiously in those suffering from hypothermia due to other causes. Other severe infections, cardiac infarction and pulmonary embolism can cause an acute derangement of thermoregulatory mechanisms. The pathogenesis of hypothermia in idiopathic steatorrhoea is ill understood, but it may be due to impaired pituitary function.[22] Accidental hypothermia occurs in patients suffering from the skin diseases psoriasis, ichthyosis and erythroderma. It has been attributed to the increased transepidermal water loss from the skin which in turn leads to increased loss of heat by vaporisation.[23]

*Clinical Manifestations*. The hypothermic patient usually has a grey appearance due to a mixture of pallor and cyanosis. The skin is cold to touch not only in exposed parts of the body but also in those parts normally covered, for example the axillae and abdominal wall. The patient often has a puffy facial appearance with slow cerebration and a husky voice which may be mistaken for myxoedema. In the absence of myxoedema these features clear when the patient recovers. Below 35°C there is some muscular weakness and incoordination and the mental state is one of dulling with diminished response to the environment. Drowsiness gives way to increasing stupor when the body temperature falls below 32°C. Consciousness is often lost when the deep body temperature is approximately 27°C and an involuntary flapping tremor of the arms and legs has been observed in some patients.[17] In the elderly the shivering reaction is not a feature of the onset of hypothermia as it may be in younger adults; even when present it disappears altogether at deep body temperatures below 32°C and is replaced by a marked increase in muscle tone leading to rigidity of the limbs and neck stiffness.

The heart rate slows in response to cold due to sinus bradycardia or to slow atrial fibrillation. The electrocardiogram usually shows some degree of heart block with an increase of the PR interval (in patients with sinus rhythm) and there is delay in intraventricular conduction. A pathognomonic sign is the appearance of a 'J' wave shown by a characteristic deflection at the junction of the QRS and ST segment.[24,25] Failure of peripheral vasoconstriction and a decrease in cardiac output lead to a fall in arterial blood pressure. This is an ominous sign. The respirations are slow and shallow, and an appreciable fall in arterial oxygen saturation may occur as a result of this hypopnoea; the effect of anoxia on the tissue metabolism is one of the factors determining prognosis.[26] Bronchopneumonia is nearly always present but it may not be detected clinically owing to the absence of the usual physical signs. Acute pancreatitis is also often present in severe hypothermia and this condition too is rarely detected. The clouding of consciousness and the muscular rigidity of the abdominal wall due to hypothermia obscure the usual signs, but pancreatitis should be suspected if the patient is seen to wince when firm pressure is applied to the epigastrium.

*Diagnosis*. The recognition of accidental hypothermia requires a high degree of awareness on the part of the physician. It should be suspected in old people who live in cold conditions even though they do not complain of feeling cold. The development of hypothermia is unassociated with symptoms and in those old people who have poor temperature discrimination there is a lack of awareness of the cold environment. Moreover, mental confusion either pre-existent or associated with hypothermia leads to difficulty in obtaining an adequate history and makes clinical examination difficult. When the condition is suspected by the finding of a low surface temperature in the normally covered parts of the body and by an oral temperature of less than 35°C the diagnosis should be confirmed by the use of a low-reading clinical thermometer placed in the rectum for five minutes. The elucidation of the underlying cause also presents difficulties, especially when it is due to hypothyroidism, diabetes mellitus, bronchopneumonia, myocardial infarction and a lesion in the central nervous system. In the absence of an obvious cause, particularly in the comatose patient, the urine and plasma should be screened for the presence of hypnotics, phenothiazine tranquillisers and anti-depressant drugs.

*Proposals for Action*

Although the number of deaths from hypothermia in old people living at home is not precisely known, the relatively large numbers of old people admitted to hospital with deep body temperatures of less than 35°C is a matter of grave concern. Until the early 1960s accidental hypothermia was comparatively common in young infants and was to be attributed to the imperfect development of thermoregulatory function in the first few weeks of life. This condition is now rarely seen and credit for its elimination has been due to public health measures instituted by community nurses. The numerically greater problem of hypothermia in old age now demands our urgent attention. In the present state of knowledge we are unable to prevent or influence the age-related decline in thermoregulatory function or the impairment of temperature discrimination. The Camden studies[11,21] have shown that diminished thermoregulatory capacity may occur in about half the elderly population. The techniques we now employ to investigate vasomotor control are complicated and there is an urgent need for physiologists to develop more simple tests for identifying this physiological disorder of function, for the individuals so affected are especially at risk. There is also a need for simpler techniques for the detection of impaired temperature discrimination which in the older person is associated with an inability to recognise a cold environment. Until these techniques are developed and we are able to recognise an 'at risk' group, measures for the prevention of hypothermia must be applied to all older people even though half the elderly population may have normal thermoregulatory function.

The studies of the Camden volunteers[21] have shown that at least two-thirds of elderly people at home suffer from medical disorders, many of which are responsible either directly or indirectly for an increased risk of hypothermia. The majority of these disorders are at present unrecognised, yet they can often be ameliorated.[27] Particular attention must be paid to the detection of postural hypotension which is often associated with impaired thermoregulatory function as well as increased liability to fall.[28] Other disorders associated with greater risk of falling are visual impairment, labyrinthine disturbances, cervical spondylosis, Parkinsonism, arthritis of the knees and postural instability associated with the use of many psychotropic drugs. It is also important to detect the endocrine disorders myxoedema and diabetes mellitus; the diagnosis of these conditions must usually depend on the results of laboratory investigations.

The housebound, who account for 8-10 per cent of old people living at home, constitute the largest group at risk. Moreover, social isolation is much more common in the housebound and the complaint of loneliness is much more frequent in this group than in the elderly population as a whole.[29] Thus the physical and mental disorders in old age which are responsible for the housebound state not only affect the mode of living and social relationships of those afflicted, but many of them are also associated with disorders of thermoregulation. Since the majority of the housebound are already known by the health and social services, the opportunities for instituting preventive measures in this group should be greater than in other vulnerable groups of old people who are not so readily identifiable. Nevertheless we still require major programmes for the early ascertainment and prevention of disability in old age involving the co-ordinated efforts of general practitioners, community nurses, social workers and the staff of hospital geriatric departments.

The best opportunities for prevention lie in the correction of the adverse social and domestic circumstances which lead the majority of old people to live in conditions which are too cold in winter. The present state in which 10 per cent of the elderly population are on the borderline of hypothermia with deep body temperatures below 35.5°C may be likened to a series of cold shocks imposed upon the individual with impaired thermoregulatory capacity and some of these are severe enough to produce true hypothermia. Priority must be given to measures which will help to ensure that elderly people are not precluded by lack of money from obtaining living conditions adequate to protect them from the cold. The majority of cases of hypothermia are due to cold exposure in the home and there is need for greater attention to improving space heating and the thermal insulation of clothing. Ideally the older person should be adequately protected to make safe forays out of doors from a warm base.

Research into the prevention of hypothermia in old age has been neglected. The younger individual successfully adapts his environment to protect himself against hazards by provision of warmth, clothing and shelter; even if these measures fail his efficient bodily thermoregulation prevents him from developing hypothermia except under conditions of extreme cold exposure. For the benefit of old people there is a need to extend this capacity for adaptation by an active approach to what might be called technological thermoregulation to replace the defective physiological thermoregulation. Would it be possible to devise clothing material with varying heat insulating properties, so that the heat flow through the material is inversely proportional to the external temperature? Such a material could be used to prevent excessive heat loss from the body surface in those individuals having impaired physiological control of heat flow from the body core to shell. There is a need too for research into suitable warning systems. Techniques are already available to monitor physical activities of old people living alone at home and the inputs to the warning systems should be extended to detect low room and body temperatures.

While awaiting these developments much could be achieved by more effective publicity to ensure that the elderly and those responsible for their welfare know about the many measures already available to meet their needs. A campaign similar to that instituted by the National Association for Maternal and Child Welfare which has eliminated infant hypothermia during the last ten years is required to reduce the magnitude of the problem of hypothermia in old age. The influence of the reports by the Royal College of Physicians[14,15] and by the British Medical Association[30] cannot readily be assessed, but certainly there is now much greater awareness by the medical and nursing professions of the hazards of a cold environment and low-reading clinical thermometers are now more widely used by general practitioners and community nurses.

## References


1. Fox. R.H., Woodward, P.M., Exton-Smith, A.N., Green, M.F., Donnison, D.V., and Wicks, M.H. (1973) 'Body Temperatures in the Elderly. A National Study of Physiological, Social and Environmental Conditions', *Brit. Med. J., 1,* 200-6
2. Edholm, O.G. (1978) *Man – Hot and Cold*, Studies in Biology No. 97, Edward Arnold, London
3. Fox, R.H. (1974) 'Temperature Regulation with Special Reference to Man' in R.J. Linden (ed.), *Recent Advances in Physiology*, Churchill Livingstone, London
4. Krag, C.L., and Kountz, W.B. (1950) 'Stability of Body Function in the Elderly. 1. Effect of Exposure of the Body to Cold', *J. Gerontol., 5,* 227-35
5. Macmillan, A.L., Corbett, J.L., Johnson, R.H., Crampton Smith, A., Spalding, J.M.K., and Wollner, L. (1967) 'Temperature Regulation in Survivors of Accidental Hypothermia of the Elderly', *Lancet, 2,* 165-9
6. Fox, R.H., Woodward, P.M., Fry, A.J., Collins, J.C., and MacDonald, I.C. (1971) 'Diagnosis of Accidental Hypothermia of the Elderly', *Lancet, 1,* 424-7
7. Department of the Environment (1977) *Homes for Today and Tomorrow*, 10th impression, HMSO, London
8. Fox, R.H. (1969) 'The Controlled Hyperthermia Heat Tolerance Test' in J.S. Weiner and J.A. Lourie *Human Biology: a Guide to Field Methods*, Blackwell, Oxford
9. Horvath, S.M. Radcliffe, C.E. Hutt, B.K., and Spurr, G.B. (1955) 'Metabolic

Responses of Old People to a Cold Environment', *J. Appt. Physiol., 8,* 145-8
10. Exton-Smith, A.N., and Overstall, P.W. (1979) *Geriatrics*, Guidelines in Medicine, vol. 1, MTP Press, Lancaster
11. Collins, K.J. Dore, C., Exton-Smith, A.N., Fox, R.H. MacDonald, I.C., and Woodward, P.M. (1977) 'Accidental Hypothermia and Impaired Temperature Homeostasis in the Elderly', *Brit. Med. J., 1,* 353-6
12. Collins, K.J., and Exton-Smith, A.N. (1980) *Urban Hypothermia: Thermoregulation, Thermal Perception and Thermal Comfort in the Elderly* (in press)
13. Rose, G., and Barker, D.J.P. (1978) 'What is a Case? Dichotomy or Continuum?', *Brit. Med. J., 2,* 873-4
14. Royal College of Physicians of London (1966) *Report of the Committee on Accidental Hypothermia*
15. Goldman, A., Exton-Smith, A.N., Francis, G., and O'Brien, A. (1977) 'A Pilot Study of Low Body Temperatures of Old People Admitted to Hospital', *J. Roy. Coll. Physcns., 11,* 291-306
16. Duguid, H., Simpson, R.G., and Stowers, J.M.(1961) 'Accidental Hypothermia', *Lancet, 2,* 1213-19
17. Rosin, A.J., and Exton-Smith, A.N. (1964) 'Clinical Features of Accidental Hypothermia, with Some Observations on Thyroid Function', *Brit. Med. J., 1,* 16-19
18. MacLean, D., and Emslie-Smith, D. (1977) *Accidental Hypothermia*, Blackwell, Oxford
19. Ewing, D.J., Campbell, I.W., and Clarke, B.F. (1976) 'Mortality in Diabetic Autonomic Neuropathy', *Lancet, 1,* 601-3
20. Phillip, G., and Smith, J.F. (1973) 'Hypothermia and Wernicke's Encephalopathy', *Lancet, 2,* 122-4
21. Exton-Smith, A.N. (1977) *The Prospects for a Long and Healthy Life*, Marjory Warren Memorial Lecture
22. Dent, C.E., Stokes, J.F., and Carpenter, M.F. (1961) 'Death from Hypothermia in Steatorrhoea', *Lancet, 1,* 748-9
23. Grice, K.A. and Bettley, F.R. (1967) 'Skin Water Loss and Accidental Hypothermia in Psoriasis, Ichthyosis and Erythroderma', *Brit. Med. J., 4,* 195-8
24. Osborn, J.J. (1953) 'Experimental Hypothermia: Respiratory and Blood pH Changes in Relation to Cardiac Function', *Amer. J. Physiol., 175,* 389-98
25. Emslie-Smith, D. (1958) 'Accidental Hypothermia: a Common Condition with a Pathognomonic ECG', *Lancet, 2,* 492-5
26. McNicol, M.W., and Smith, R. (1964) 'Accidental Hypothermia', *Brit. Med. J., 1,* 19-21
27. Williamson, J., Stokoe, I.H., Gray, S., Fisher, M., Smith, A., McGhee, A., and Stephenson, E. (1964) 'Old People at Home – their Unreported Needs', *Lancet, 1,* 1117-20
28. Overstall, P.W., Exton-Smith, A.N., Imms, F.J., and Johnson, A.L. (1977) 'Falls in the Elderly Related to Postural Imbalance', *Brit. Med. J., 1,* 261-4
29. Sheldon, J.H. (1948) *The Social Medicine of Old Age*, Oxford University Press, Oxford
30. British Medical Association (1964) 'Accidental Hypothermia in the Elderly', *Brit. Med. J., 2,* 1255-8

# 4 PARKINSONISM AND AGEING*

Donald B. Calne

## Age-related Changes and Parkinsonism

Many diseases become increasingly common with advancing age. Degenerative disorders such as osteoarthritis and atherosclerosis are examples. In addition, neoplasia is more frequently encountered in the elderly, and the incidence of infective illness is high, presumably because of deteriorating immunological responses. The mere correlation of disease incidence or prevalence with late life does not, therefore, cast any light on aetiology. However, there are some features of Parkinsonism (Figure 4.1) which merit special consideration in this context. The most notable point is that in many ways the syndrome of Parkinsonism represents a caricature of the popular image of getting old (Figure 4.2). The patient typically has a stooped posture, slow movements, a shuffling gait, tremulous hands and some dulling of intellectual activity. The traditional painting, sculpture or literary description of age embodies all these features. Could it be that Parkinsonism is a natural consequence of ageing in the nervous system, just as wrinkling of the skin and greying of the hair signal ageing of the integument? Put another way, can the population be divided simply into those who have Parkinsonism and those who are going to get it unless they die from another cause first? There is no answer to this question yet, although relevant evidence is beginning to accrue.

Many age-related changes have been thought to be exaggerated in Parkinsonism. At a morphological level it has been reported that neurons in the substantia nigra accumulate lipofuscin, lose melanin, and die with the passage of time; but the depletion of nigral cells is especially marked in Parkinsonism[1] (Figure 4.3). Dopamine is the neurotransmitter employed by the zona compacta cells of the substantia nigra, and the concentration of this amine falls in late life,[2] with a substantial accentuation of this loss in Parkinsonism.[3] Similar relationships to ageing and Parkinsonism have been established for tyrosine hydroxylase,[1] the enzyme responsible for the rate limiting step in the synthesis of dopamine, and for tetrahydrobiopterin (THB), its co-

*This chapter was written by the author in his private capacity. No official support nor endorsement is intended or should be inferred.

**Figure 4.1: Age specific Prevalence Rates per 100,000 Population for Parkinsonism: Rochester, Minnesota, 1 January 1954**

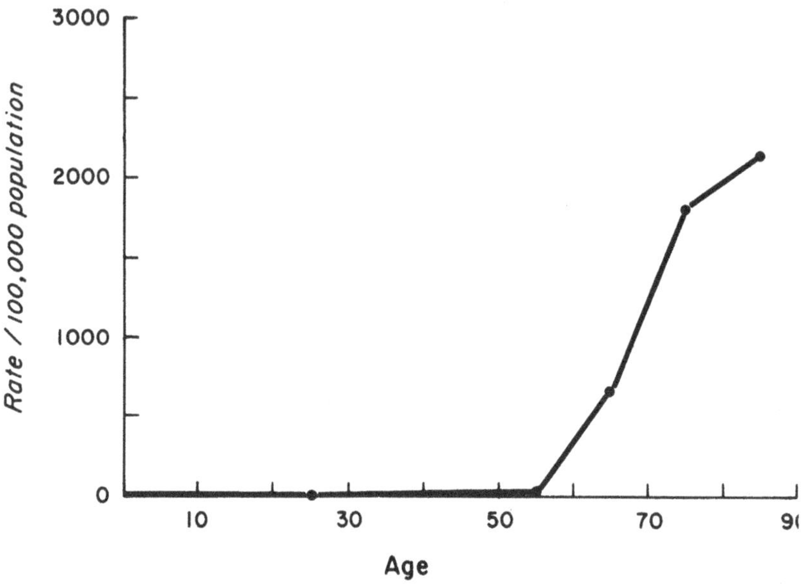


Source: L.T. Kurland, J.F. Kurtzke and I.D. Goldberg, *Epidemiology of Neurologic and Sense Organ Disorders* Harvard University Press, Cambridge, Mass., 1973, p. 55. Reprinted by permission.

factor[4] (Figures 4.4 and 4.5).

Finally, a number of clinical features of ageing of the nervous system are either more frequent or more severe in Parkinsonism;[5] posture, slowing of movement, tremor and dementia have already been mentioned. Other examples include paresis of ocular convergence, constipation and impairment of balance. However, in interpreting these observations there are certain pitfalls, such as whether the reduction of THB in the cerebrospinal fluid (CSF) represents a biochemical index of premature or accelerated ageing which might be relevant to the aetiology of Parkinsonism.

As already mentioned, THB is a cofactor for tyrosine hydroxylase, the enzyme responsible for the rate limiting step in dopamine synthesis. The concentration of THB in the CSF falls with age (Figure 4.5), but in patients with Parkinson's disease the level is even lower than that of age-matched controls (Figure 4.6). From these observations it might

**Figure 4.2: Parkinson's Disease**

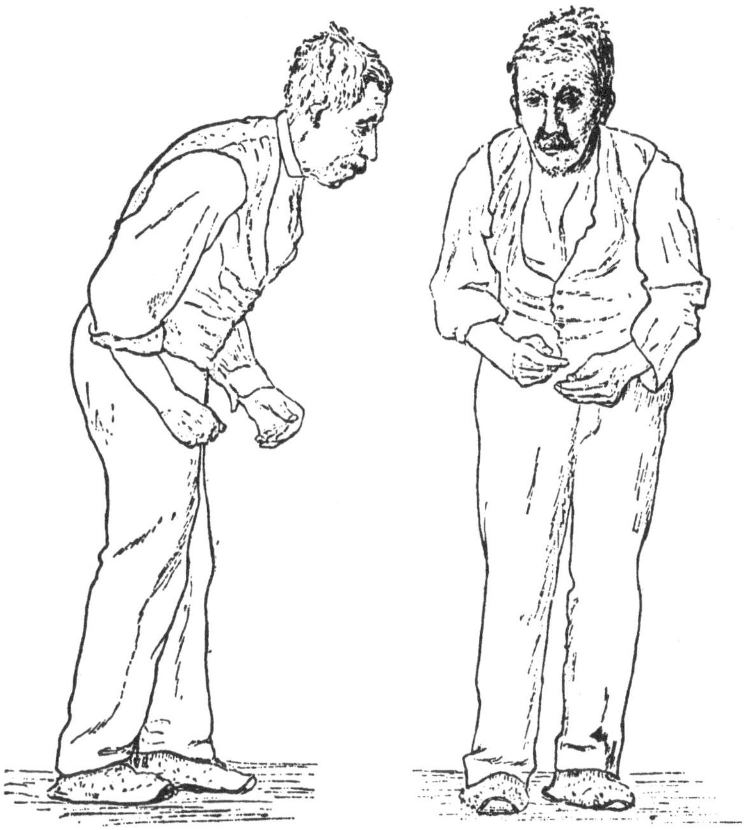

Source: W.R. Gowers, *A Manual of Diseases of the Nervous System* J. and A. Churchill, London, 1893), vol. II, p. 639 (after St Leger).

be inferred that a reduction of THB is a marker for Parkinsonism, possibly reflecting the loss of neurons from the substantia nigra, or even providing a clue to aetiology. As such, the THB concentration would be of considerable interest as a biochemical index of nigral disease which could be evaluated in man prior to death. Further studies have shown that depletion of THB in the CSF occurs in several diseases of the nervous system[6] (Figure 4.7). This refutation of specificity attributable to the THB changes excludes any possibility that reduced cofactor plays an aetiological role in Parkinsonism, though it is still in accord with the THB loss representing death of monoaminergic neurons. The

**Figure 4.3: Cell Counts in Substantia Nigra of Humans Plotted against Age**

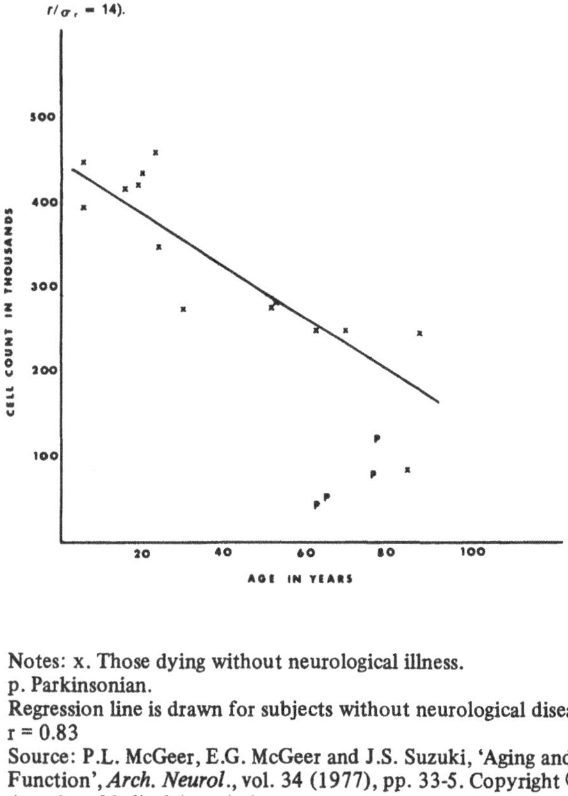


Notes: x. Those dying without neurological illness.
p. Parkinsonian.
Regression line is drawn for subjects without neurological disease.
r = 0.83
Source: P.L. McGeer, E.G. McGeer and J.S. Suzuki, 'Aging and Extrapyramidal Function', *Arch. Neurol.*, vol. 34 (1977), pp. 33-5. Copyright © 1977, American Medical Association.

evolution of information on THB illustrates the dangers of over-interpreting the significance of abnormalities of any kind found in Parkinsonism. Up to now, the only deficit that the overwhelming weight of evidence supports as central to the functional disturbances of Parkinson's disease is the depletion of dopamine in the striatum, with the associated loss of the nigrostriatal neuronal projection.

While it is evident that studies of the relationship of Parkinsonism to age have not led to any important advance in our understanding of aetiology, there remain some curious observations which may shed light on the problem at some future date. For example, levodopa extends the life expectation of Hale-Stoner mice, which commonly die young from

**Figure 4.4: Calculated Curve of Tyrosine Hydroxylase Activity as Function of Age in Caudate and Putamen of Humans Dying without Neurological Illness**

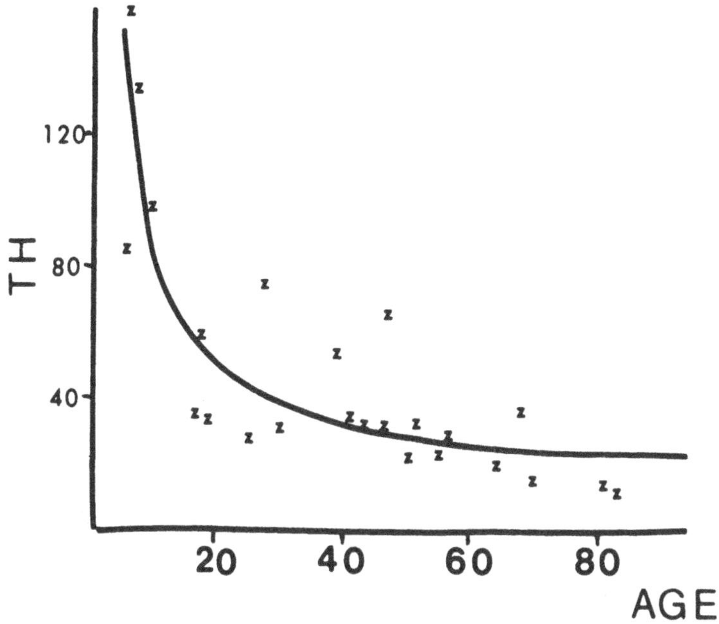


Note: Measurements for tyrosine hydroxylase in nanomoles per hour per 100 mg of protein.
Source: McGeer *et al.*, 'Aging and Extrapyramidal Function'.

various degenerations involving the central nervous system.[7] Similarly, chronic toxicological studies with the dopaminergic agent bromocriptine have revealed a tendency for moderate doses of this drug to lengthen life in rats, and another dopaminergic drug, lergotrile, has been shown to restore oestrus in elderly female rats.[8] In a recent study, elderly rats have been found to display a characteristic deficit in swimming: they lack vigour and are less capable of keeping their heads above water. Administration of levodopa, or the dopaminergic drug apomorphine, reverses this age-related disability.[9]

These observations cannot be woven into a pattern sufficiently coherent to form the basis of an explanation of the role of dopaminergic mechanisms in the ageing brain, but they do pose some tantalising

**Figure 4.5: Hydroxylase Cofactor Activity as a Function of Age**

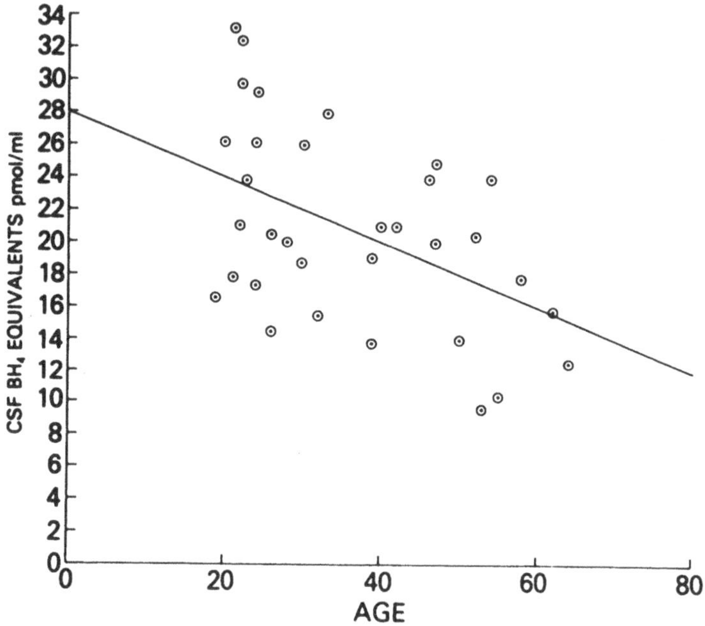


Source: R.A. Levine, A.C. Williams, D.S. Robinson, D.B. Calne and W. Lovenberg, 'Analysis of Hydroxylase Cofactor Activity in the Cerebrospinal Fluid of Patients with Parkinson's Disease' in L.J. Poirier, T.L. Sourkes and P.J. Bedard (eds.), *Advances in Neurology, vol. 24. The Extrapyramidal System and its Disorders* (Raven Press, New York, 1979), pp. 303-7.

enigmas. At a time when the precursors of neurotransmitters are becoming fashionable as dietary adjuvants, one might even speculate whether it is remotely possible that long-term intake of low doses of levedopa might be a plausible if eccentric approach to some of the problems of normal neurological ageing.

Before passing on to consider some more practical aspects of the diagnosis and management of Parkinson's disease, it is perhaps permissible to comment on some general aspects of the ageing process. Finch[10] has stressed the importance of the co-ordinating mechanisms of the body in sustaining general vitality. A breakdown in the controlling forces exercised by the nervous, endocrine and immune systems can be anticipated to produce a catastrophic decline in the ability of the organism to adjust to a changing external and internal environment, and

**Figure 4.6: Hydroxylase Cofactor in Normal and Parkinsonian Patients**

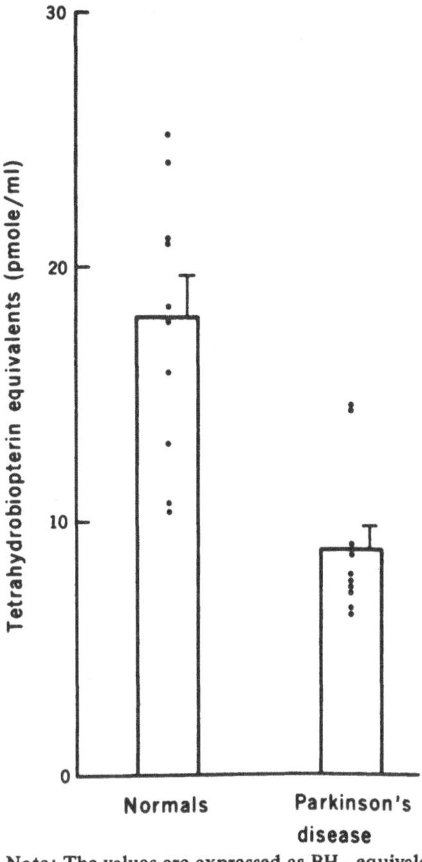


Note: The values are expressed as $BH_4$ equivalents. Each data point represents the mean of samples assayed in triplicate. All patients gave their informed consent to this study. Lumbar punctures were done at 9 a.m. after all patients had been at bed rest for 8 hours and had only a standard low monoamine diet for 48 hours. A series of 2-ml portions of CSF were collected, frozen by the bedside in dry ice, and then quickly transferred for storage in liquid nitrogen.
Source: W. Lovenberg, R.A. Levine, D.S. Robinson, M. Ebert, A.C. Williams and D.B. Calne, 'Hydroxylase Cofactor Activity in Cerebrospinal Fluid of Normal Subjects and Patients with Parkinson's Disease', *Science*, vol. 204 (1979), pp. 624-6.

to deal with such inevitable problems as exposure to infective agents, the occurrence of deleterious mutations, the avoidance of physically undesirable surroundings and, in the case of man, the solution of new cognitive tasks. Failure to cope in any of these areas is likely to lead to

**Figure 4.7: Hydroxylase Cofactor Levels in the Lumbar CSF of Patients with Some Neurological Diseases**

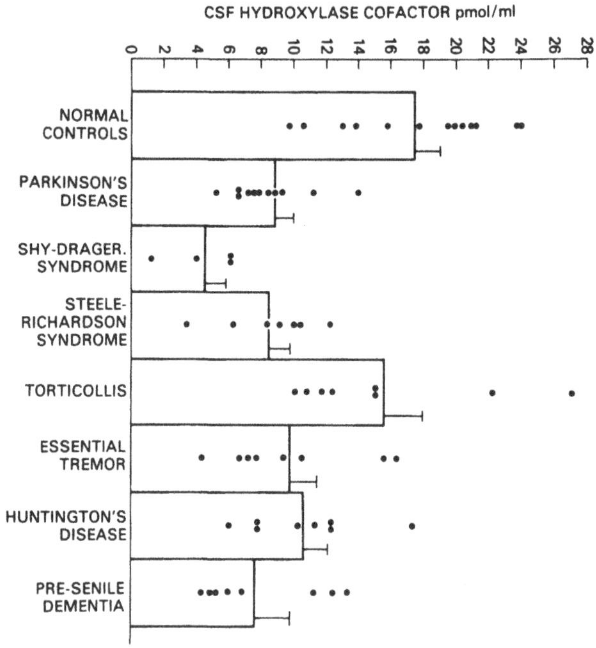


Note: The mean values and standard errors for each group are indicated.
Source: A.C. Williams, R.A. Levine, D.B. Calne, T.N. Chase and W. Lovenberg, 'CSF Hydroxylase Cofactor Levels in Some Neurological Diseases' (1980) (in preparation).

a cascade of non-specific problems which, taken together, might perhaps be construed to comprise those disorders that distinguish 'geriatric' patients from the rest of adult medicine.

Mortality increases exponentially after maturity, and it is a cold, discomforting feature of natural selection that there does not seem to be any biological advantage in survival of parents after the offspring have established their independence. Indeed, since resources are limited, it can be argued that nature must ensure disappearance of the post-mature to allow the young to develop and in turn reproduce. Here is the teleological explanation of biological deterioration with advancing age. In attempting to alleviate pain and extend life all physicians are fighting these harsher aspects of nature, but the geriatrician's wits are pitted against much greater odds than his colleagues, because senescence presents such a vicious circle of declining resistance to disease. While life may be terminated by failure in a specific vital organ, there is more often an incomplete widespread degeneration of many components, any of which might be connected individually, but which collectively result in a loss of homeostatic capability and death from relatively trivial causes.

Just as the organism, as a whole, is made up of a myriad of independently ageing elements, each organ possesses components which undergo senescence at different rates. In the brain, cell dysfunction is especially poignant because neurons cannot replicate. It is easy to demonstrate, for example, that the vestibular nuclei survive ageing better than the substantia nigra, and correspondingly some neurotransmitters (such as acetylcholine, gamma-aminobutyric acid (GABA), glycine and glutamate) persist through senescence more readily than others (such as dopamine and norepinephrine).

In examining the aetiology of disease in the elderly, the concept of normality must first be considered. The term 'normal' is usually employed to describe any feature that occurs in the majority of subjects, so it is in this sense correct to regard a number of clinical deficits in the elderly as normal (although these may be undesirable and differ from healthy young adults). By this usage, normal senescence merges into pathological ageing, in which deterioration of function ultimately leads to death. Others reserve the term 'normal' for subjects that are free of pathology, irrespective of age. From this semantic controversy, the problem of the aetiology of Parkinsonism re-emerges; does this disease represent premature ageing or senescence plus a specific neuropathological entity? Since rare cases of juvenile Parkinsonism occur, it seems more likely that the idiopathic condition derives from an extraneous infective or biochemical disturbance, rather than exacerbation of a non-specific ageing process which is taking place in the brain.

## Diagnosis and Management of Parkinsonism

The diagnosis of advanced Parkinsonism is straightforward, but early disease can be difficult to identify, especially in patients over 70 years of age, when slow movement, poor balance and impairment of memory are common. Senile tremor may also be difficult to distinguish from

Parkinsonism, although it usually has a prominent action component.

The treatment of Parkinsonism also poses special problems in the elderly. These comprise:

(1) variation in dose-response relationships, because of altered pharmacokinetics – slower absorption, slower metabolism, slower excretion, smaller volume of distribution;
(2) more drug interactions, because elderly patients are often taking a complex compendium of medications for multiple disorders;
(3) more adverse reactions, because concomitant diseases lower the threshold for such unwanted drug effects as confusion, hypotension and, in men, urinary retention;
(4) reduced compliance, because elderly patients are less consistent in taking their medication; this difficulty can sometimes be overcome by suitable surveillance by the family.

Current treatment for Parkinsonism is undergoing reappraisal following the recognition of difficult management problems, such as increasing dyskinesia, psychiatric reactions and on-off phenomena, all of which tend to develop after a substantial cumulative dose of levodopa. Now many neurologists start newly diagnosed patients on anticholinergic drugs or amantadine, keeping levodopa until it really becomes necessary, and then giving in the minimum dose required to achieve an adequate therapeutic response. The decision when to start levodopa, and what constitutes an adequate therapeutic response, will depend on the social, economic and psychological resources of the patient and often the extent of unrelated disease. It is relevant, for example, that Parkinsonian tremor is largely a cosmetic problem, causing more embarrassment than functional disability. By far the most important indications for levodopa are declining general mobility and bulbar involvement. If patients have previously been taking levodopa without a peripheral decarboxylase inhibitor, there is no need to modify their regimen unless they are experiencing those adverse effects which might be improved by extra-cerebral blockade of decarboxylase (emesis, cardiac arrhythmias, angle-closure glaucoma). Patients to be started on levodopa have everything to gain and nothing to lose by taking it in combination with a decarboxylase inhibitor such as carbidopa (in Sinemet) or benserazide (in Madopar).

Recent studies indicate that some patients who encounter prominent dyskinesia or on-off reactions may improve with a reduction of levodopa and addition of bromocriptine, a direct dopamine agonist.[11] However, special caution is desirable if bromocriptine is given to old people, since it can precipitate severe schizophrenic reactions. Dosage should be considerably lower than that given routinely for Parkinson's disease.

Surgery is seldom undertaken now for Parkinsonism. Stereotactic lesions of the contralateral ventrolateral nucleus of the thalamus usually alleviate tremor, but they can also induce permanent neurological deficits, particularly when operative procedures are bilateral, and have to be repeated.

In addition to pharmacotherapy and surgery, it is desirable to sustain the patient's morale with encouragement, pursuit of hobbies, occupational therapy, formation of self-help associations with other patients, and any additional measures that will keep the patient physically and mentally active. Physical therapy is often rewarding, particularly for patients who have lost their confidence in walking. Discussions between the physician and the family may be as important for the patient as the prescription of medications. Commonly the spouse or child is playing a crucial supportive role which may require guidance, and always benefits from reinforcement and reaffirmation of its value.

## Conclusions

Parkinson's disease has an intriguing but still obscure relationship with the general process of ageing of the nervous system. Diagnosis of early disease can be tricky, and management will test the skill of the physician as a clinical pharmacologist, co-ordinator of support services and family adviser. Few diseases provide the medical practitioner, and particularly the geriatric neurologist, with such a demanding and rewarding mix of academic and practical challenges.

## References

1. McGeer, P.L., McGeer, E.G., and Suzuki, J.S. (1977) 'Aging and Extra-pyramidal Function', *Arch. Neurol., 34,* 33-5
2. Carlsson, A., and Winblad, B. (1976) 'Influence of Age and Time Interval between Death and Autopsy on Dopamine and 3-methoxytyramine Levels in Human Basal Ganglia', *J. Neural Trans., 38*, 271-6
3. Hornykiewicz, O. (1966) 'Dopamine (3-hydroxytyramine) and Brain Function', *Pharmacol. Rev., 181,* 925-64
4. Levine, R.A. Williams, A.C., Robinson, D.S., Calne, D.B., and Lovenberg, W. (1979) 'Analysis of Hydroxylase Cofactor Activity in the Cerebrospinal Fluid of Patients with Parkinson's Disease' in L.J. Poirier, T.L. Sourkes and P.J.

Bedard (eds.), *Advances in Neurology, vol. 24. The Extrapyramidal System and its Disorders*, Raven Press, New York pp. 303-7

5. Barbeau, A. (1973) 'Aging and the Extrapyramidai System', *J. Am. Geriatr. Soc., 21*, 145-9
6. Williams, A.C., Levine, R.A., Calne, D.B., Chase, T.N., and Lovenberg, W. (1980) 'CSF Hydroxylase Cofactor Levels in Some Neurological Diseases', *J. Neurol. Neurosurg. Psychiatry*, in press
7. Cotzias, G.C., Miller, S.T., Nicholson, A.R., Maston, W.H., and Tang, L.C. (1974) 'Prolongation of the Life-span in Mice Adapted to Large Amounts of L-dopa', *Proc. Nat. Acad. Sci., 71*, 2466-9
8. Clemens, J.A., and Bennett, D.E. (1977) 'Do Aging Changes in the Preoptic Area Contribute to Loss of Cyclic Endocrine Function?' *J. Gerontol., 32*, 19-24
9. Marshall, J.F., and Berrios, N. (1979) 'Movement Disorders of Aged Rats: Reversal by Dopamine Receptor Stimulation', *Science, 206*, 477-9
10. Finch, C.E. (1976) 'The Regulation of Physiological Changes during Mammalian Aging', *Q. Rev. Biol., 51*, 49-83
11. Calne, D.B., Williams, A.C., Neophytides, A., Plotkin, C., Nutt, J.G., and Teychenne, P.F. (1978) 'Long-term Treatment of Parkinsonism with Bromocriptine', *Lancet, 1*, 735-7

# PART TWO: PSYCHIATRY

# 5 DEMENTIA: MISFITS IN NEED OF CARE

David Jolley

## Introduction

Most lives are free and private. Babies and infants are dependent on mother and close family for care and supervision, but this is a transitional state. Maturation and practice bring the abilities to sit, crawl, walk, talk and think. These skills provide the opportunity for secret and personal activity, a source of pride, pleasure and sometimes pain to parents. Some will choose to spend their lives in fond closeness with loved ones, others will be more determined in the search for and defence of independence. All will choose how much of their lives to share, with whom and when. Attempts to breach the circle of self, or the territory that becomes identified with it, promote rapid and violent response in all but the most pliant. Self-reliance is highly prized by individuals themselves and by society.

There are situations where it is acceptable that barriers will be lowered and others allowed in. Such is the basis of loving relationships and at times of particular vulnerability, such as illness, certain professional groups, including doctors, nurses and the clergy, have gained licence to intrude for a while to perform necessary tasks.

At a gross level the attainment of selfhood and privacy is reflected in living circumstances. Thus children live with parents but then pass through a series of situations with progressively less dependence on others, culminating usually in old age where for the first time living alone is common. Thus one can trace a thread of progressive independence and self-reliance associated with gaining a greater age. Yet a second contrary and pathological thread takes 3 per cent of 65-74-year-olds away from private households into institutions and this loss of private status rises to 8 per cent of 75-84-year-olds and 21 per cent of those over 85 years.[1,2]

While most old people choose to live in the house occupied during their working lives a few seek the advantages (real or imagined) of seaside resorts and an increasing number are 'corralled' into 'more suitable' flats or bungalows. Even among those old people who persist in their own homes some will surrender their privacy as home helps, meals on wheels, health visitors, district nurses and others gain regular access to the most secret of times and activities.

There is a sense in which this is shocking and seems to be shameful. What kind of society is it that treats its elderly by locking them away or riding roughshod over their hard-earned dignity! The lives of elderly people are public concern, public property.

A number of factors are responsible for the frailty and vulnerability of very old people. Probably the most important is the accumulation of disease processes – old and new in the aged body. Among these the dementias alone or in combination with other illnesses produce the greatest erosion of the ability for self-reliance and place the sufferer in the hands of others.

## Mental Disorders of Late Life

The concept of dementia is well established in psychiatric thinking since the descriptive writings on old age by the ancients have given way to the systematic clinical analyses of the German alienists of the nineteenth century.[3] Yet the differontiation of the dementias from other psychotic states in late life has not always been maintained and our present generation owes a great debt to Dr Felix Post for his meticulous clinical contributions and Sir Martin Roth for analyses of larger groups.[4,5] These have reaffirmed that depressive states are common among the elderly presented to mental hospitals. Many are treatable with modern therapies and, though some people continue to suffer symptoms on a chronic or recurrent basis, most require relatively little in the way of support from statutory services[6] and their life expectation is only modestly reduced.[7]

Paranoid states are seen less frequently, but arouse great interest. A few people presenting with paranoid ideas deteriorate over a period and appear to be suffering from dementing illnesses, but most lose their paranoid ideas with modern medicines[8] and their well preserved if atypical personalities allow them to persist in a stylised independence.

The dementias are also common among the elderly presented to psychiatrists. Their clinical characteristics have remained the same over the years and sadly no specific medication nor other manipulation has emerged to modify the range of management that can be offered.

These important and well described mental disorders seen by psychiatrists are by no means confined to mental hospitals. A number of surveys of old people at home have identified mood disorders a-plenty, paranoid disorders more rarely, but dementias in 5-10 per cent.[9,10,11,12] It seems probable that many of the depressive states not known to services are 'neurotic' or 'reactive', for some people find it very difficult to live with the stresses and responsibilities that are peculiar to old age. They find themselves in a time and territory that was not explored by their parents and are viewed by much of society as alienated. Outside the work culture, non-contributory, they are a liability to those who create wealth, as they are heavy consumers of entertainment and supportive services. Many self-possessed people find it devastating to find themselvės unable through their own efforts or self-sacrifice to care for themselves or maintain their care of others. The neurotic conflicts of late life are now presented in bulk – yet our understanding of them, particularly in the climate produced by such a large old age population, is rudimentary.

Klaus Bergmann has pioneered the way,[13] taking off from epidemiological research and stimulating Alistair McKechnie to carry on.[14] Much will be gained by further efforts, perhaps linked with a greater awareness of the place of old people in society and expansion of gerontological research and education.

Set alongside the new growth of interest in neurotic disorders of late life, the dementias are gnarled old wood and are of a different order. They produce easily identified gross impairment of function, the nature of which has been known to generations. A mental illness that all would deem psychotic, this is not the stuff for the analyst's couch nor the academic clinic. It is coarse and bludgeoning in its destruction and shameless in its demand for service of the crudest, most engulfing kind. Words, medicines, sophisticated investigations are puny and often irrelevant; time, organised old-fashioned care by resourceful people in appropriate buildings are effective. Yet these are scarce, expensive and undervalued.

## The Syndrome of Dementia

Dementia is in itself a term that has frightened or depressed people so much that there has evolved a range of alternatives for professional or lay usage. This is unfortunate, as every alternative terminology demands investigation and understanding if productive conversations are to take place between users. In practice, such comparative exercises have not been undertaken and the issues that surround 'dementia' escape confrontation.

As Lishman[15] explains: 'dementia' is a thoroughly respectable word and can be used to describe a syndrome characterised as 'an acquired global impairment of memory and personality but without impairment of consciousness'. This syndrome may be produced by a number of pathologies of variable progress. In addition, a number of 'disease entities' – 'dementing illnesses' are accommodated within the syndrome but currently share an expectation of inevitable deterioration and early death.

Within the memory disorder, loss of ability with recent information is crudely obvious to all observers, but systematic studies confirm family comments that recall from distant memory stores is also faulty. At the same time, sometimes out of proportion to the memory decline, initiative declines and quantity and quality of constructive activity are rapidly compromised. This is most easily appreciated in an interview, where speech may be difficult to elicit or unproductive with frequent repetitions of favoured stories and anecdotes of the past or limited and facile preoccupation with details of the present. On the broader canvas of life at home, the proud gardener may have been overgrown by the seasons which bring new crops whether attended or not. The proud housekeeper may be cluttered or the cupboard bare as omissions of discharge or recharge predominate. Activity and conversation are stultified, stereotyped and repetitive. Thus within a limited circle of waking, drinking tea with bread and butter, laying utensils aside unwashed until used again, a passable competence may obtain, but making plans for a balanced and interesting diet through major shopping expeditions that take account of tomorrow and the next day become a thing of the past. A chat about the weather, general health matters or mild reminiscences of well loved events allow a nodding approach to conversation, enjoyable in itself and accepted at many a public bar, bingo hall or cocktail party, but richer excursions of the mind are no longer available.

That mood which has prevailed throughout life persists, but has less flexibility and can no longer withstand so well the changes demanded by external events. So the sensitive approach paranoia, the timid become fearful, the happy-go-lucky become disinhibited and the miserable, crabby. Pressures that demand rapid change may be outside the range of graded response and an explosion of catastrophic, chaotic output is all that is possible.

This clinical syndrome can be produced by a number of recognised pathologies: space-occupying lesions within the skull, including subdural haematoma, primary and secondary malignancies, normal pressure hydrocephalus, brain injury related to trauma, infections, especially the chronic infections due to tuberculosis and neurosyphilis, toxins of various sorts, but most particularly alcohol, anoxia, vitamin deficiencies and endocrine disorders and the pharmacy.[16] A careful search for these or any of the rarer 'causes' of dementia is one task the clinician accepts readily. In some instances an appreciation of the 'causative agent' opens up possibilities for treatment with the hope of reversing or arresting the process. At other times thorough investigation may be helpful from the medico-legal point of view. Even in those situations where it is possible to identify factors such as those outlined above it is usual to find that the patient requires and continues to require management appropriate to established defective function.[17]

Among the elderly the vast majority of people presenting with a dementing syndrome are suffering from one of the two major dementing illnesses: senile dementia, which is now becoming termed 'Alzheimer's dementia', or arteriosclerotic dementia, now being termed 'multiple infarct dementia'.[18] These have in common not only the broad characteristics of the dementing syndrome, but also progressive deterioration to early death. This has been monitored in hospitalised patients[19] and community studies.[20] It is possible that the rate of progression can be predicted from features of the mental state[21] and age of the sufferer.[22] In addition, it seems probable that the absence of other, particularly physical, illnesses must be important, as is the prevailing socio-psychological situation.[23]

At the present time our understanding of the pathological processes involved is improving very impressively. Yet our ability to influence the essential course of either illness remains extremely limited. This is not to say that medication has no part to play in management, indeed medications may be used to good effect in treating a variety of symptoms arising during the course of a dementia.[24] There is even the possibility that life expectation within the dementias has been significantly increased by the availability of antibiotics.[25]

Studies in different countries concur in finding that social circumstances are not involved in the genesis of dementia,[26,27] but underline the importance of social circumstances in management.[28] The current estimates that 5 per cent of elderly at home are severely demented and another 5 per cent show milder stigmata may prove to be misleadingly reassuring when the full impact of the population explosion among septuagenarians and octogenarians is upon us.[29]

### *Senile Dementia*

This condition is characterised by a gradual progressive loss of cognitive and personality function as described above and is seen most commonly among old ladies. This is certainly because there are more old ladies than old gentlemen, and those men that survive into old age usually do so in company with a spouse who will accommodate their failings. Familial patterns are probably based on multi-factorial genetic inheritance, though in some families simple Mendelian dominance is identified.[30] Chromosomal abnormalities have been described in some female dements,[31] and increasingly fascinating links with Down's Syndrome and other chromosomal aberrations have been noted.[32] Peripheral nerve conduction is probably reduced in proportion to the severity of dementia and supports the possibility that the illness is not confined in its effects to the central nervous system.[33]

The morbid pathology and light microscope characteristics of senile dementia have been clarified by Corsellis.[34] From his work attention has been concentrated on the senile plaque and neurofibrillary tangle. Tomlinson and Blessed[35] were able to demonstrate a quantitative relationship between psychological decline and increased senile plaque count. Electron microscopy has provided further understanding of the structure of senile plaques and it seems possible that the first change to occur is the deposition of an amyloid core around which accumulates debris derived from distorted neurites. Within the neurones, neurofibrillary tangles are probably derived from neurotubules whose protein has become denatured. Despite all this disruption and the light microscopists' impression of widespread 'degeneration', there remains a good deal of normal structure within the dementing nervous system: in particular some synaptic clefts are seen to be preserved. A tentative optimism comes from the laboratories, enhanced by new biochemical findings. These have identified deficiencies of choline acetyl transferase (CAT), an enzyme essential to the production of acetyl choline.[36] The deficiency of this enzyme parallels the accumulation of senile plaques and impaired memory function recognised as the hallmarks of senile dementia.[37] An enthusiastic search is on to produce an agent capable of circumventing or correcting this biochemical fault in the hope that this may 'switch on' the neuronal substrate. Whilst all this interest and enthusiasm is uplifting, there are warnings that such a simple model of limited biochemical dysfunction may not account for all the deficiences presented in this illness. Up to the present time the only group of patients reliably improved by choline supplements have been those with motor disorders. Yet even within Parkinsonism, the only neurological condition where a similar biochemical model has been used to good effect, the improvements obtained with L-dopa are limited and may be balanced by undesirable effects and the underlying condition continues to progress. Similarly, the essence of senile dementia is already demonstrated to have broader biochemical correlates with reduced levels of ribonucleic acid in nerve cells throughout the central nervous system.[38] This may prove to be of greater significance than the CAT story.

Recently interest has been raised in the immunological status of dements and the possibility that an infective agent such as a 'slow virus' or a reactivated commensal virus is responsible for some forms of dementia is taken seriously.[39] Thus senile dementia is accepted as a disease entity rather than an inevitable consequence of growing old and is now thought of as part of a continuum which includes 'presenile' Alzheimer dementia.

### *Cerebrovascular Dementia*

Whilst there has been some difficulty in accepting senile dementia as an illness, the psychosis associated with arteriosclerosis of cerebral vessels has been more readily seen as such. The clinical course is characterised by stepwise deterioration of function associated with acute neurological incidents; dysphasia, paralysis, convulsions, etc., which usually leave identifiable sequelae. In this condition fair-sized chunks of brain tissue may be killed off, leaving the rest of the otherwise normal brain to compensate as best it may. Hypertension predisposes to arteriosclerosis and within the brain makes the creation of lacunae and areas of softening more common. In addition the arteriopath is likely to have an ischaemic heart which may produce sudden falls of blood pressure at times of coronary thrombosis or dysrhythmia and any interference with blood flow by intraluminar plaques in the carotids must aggravate such vagaries of perfusion pressure as well as adding material to the blood stream that may impact as microemboli within the cerebral end-arteries.[40] The presence of the various arteriosclerotic defects in the cerebral circulation leaves it less flexible in response to stress and this probably explains the considerable fluctuation in performance of the arteriosclerotic brain.[41] At one level the loss of ability is determined by the volume of cerebral cortex infarcted[35] and independent of CAT enzyme levels.[37] Optimal function is obtained by the best exercise of that potentially healthy tissue which remains. At the present time it seems doubtful if the cerebral vasodilators are very helpful in this task.[42] Control of blood pressure is essential in some cases and it may be that reducing platelet stickiness with aspirin or similar compounds will find an important place in therapy.

## Patterns of Care: at Home

These two forms of dementia remain essentially unresponsive to medications in this medicine-revering age. So what patterns of service have these conditions evoked, and are there any pointers towards which interventions are successful in meeting the needs of people suffering from dementia or caring for someone who does?

Most old people suffering from dementia live at home. Many men and fewer women will be living with a spouse of forty to fifty years' standing. Such couples have shared a great deal. The present generation have gone through two world wars, seen hunger marches, a revolution in transport from horses and carriages to space travel and now accept television as a day-to-day presence when their childhood could not have dreamed of such a thing. Even when a marriage has been firmly bedded in hatred, such lengthy familiarity usually carries with it a preparedness to care for the other in disability. In the folklore of growing old loss of memory and muddled-headedness are accepted as 'senility'. The older you are before it comes, the less likely is such 'symptomatology' to be dignified as 'illness'. Even the fluctuating and stepwise course of the arteriosclerotic states in very old people is accepted as 'dizzy-does' and 'queer turns' – certainly not worthy to trouble the doctor. The slow progression of dementias means that it is relatively easy for a spouse to accommodate to the escalating demands. This becomes their task, their secret, in both their interests to keep others at bay, neither wanting the ailing partner to be put away. The quality of care is almost always admirable, for the care giver is well equipped. A house shared for fifty years may lack modern conveniences but is strong in cues to memories past, and those essentials such as chair, bed, toilet and water are constantly sited. Trips to the shops can be a mutual pleasure. When bodily care becomes necessary it does not require the crossing of taboo boundaries. Thus the calm and peace of this well rehearsed complementary pairing reduces the likelihood of secondary complications such as anxiety, depression or paranoid thinking. It may require a catastrophe to disrupt the situation, but personal catastrophes are not rare among old people. They may befall the dementing or caregiving partner. Physical illness in the dementing may demand nursing beyond the skills or endurance of the spouse. Physical illness within the carer may end her ability to provide for her partner who by virtue of his dementia, cannot respond to her new needs. Social changes are also dangerous. Changes of housing, be it on a temporary basis, as for a holiday or to allow for 'improvements' to the home, or on a permanent basis to 'sheltered' housing, are notable for their potential for harm. Gone is the reassuring backcloth learned and modified over the years. Immediately relaxation is less easy, heightened arousal the order of the day and the elderly couple perform beneath their best. Changes in mental health, particularly the emergence of a depressive illness or dementia in the caring partner, provide a third dimension by which weakness may develop in the 'husband and wife co-operative'.

The husband and wife system is seen to have many ingredients of success; the trick for other caring agencies to develop in relationship to it is that of providing help without invading its self-sufficiency.

In addition, the professional and voluntary groups prepared and interested to work with elderly demented people must copy the methods demonstrated in their successful, informed caring partnership and assimilate them into their more formal care-giving operations. A number of 'treatment' strategies have been evolved recently and dignified with impressive rationale.[43] These are extremely useful but one should remain sensible of the humble achievements that common sense spawns in many homely situations whose quality of success in the management of individuals cannot be bettered. It is usually wiser to add to these natural experiments than to impose regimes based on ill-understood and less securely based dogma.

An old person alone is much more vulnerable. A life-long loner may have well developed coping abilities that survive even into a dementia. Yet those personality attributes that have kept him alone for so many years may make it difficult now to allow in those prepared to give essential services. The widowed may find it very difficult to compensate for emerging shortcomings when the experience of a life shared has carried the expectation of a corrective response from another for any waywardness.

Sisters and brothers sometimes come together again in late life. It is wonderful to see how clearly the competitions of youth are taken up as fresh as if the interlude of fifty years had never been. Inter-sib caring can be impressive, but usually falls short in quality and quantity of that demonstrated within marriages. The same can be said with more certainty of that most frequently discussed support system: daughter, especially married daughter taking on mum or dad, or an in-law. Where mother or father is failing to cope because of a dementia, a reasonable relationship can be maintained so long as the elder can be suppported by visits. For hours at a time it seems the bricks and mortar aided by furnishings cope alone. Yet disturb this secret ingredient by the best of intentions and uncertainty rides supreme. Thus a move nearer to daughter, or a move to live in her house may 'hold' for a while, but there are frequently rapid escalations in tension that are hard for either party to bear. The loss of well known surroundings, the loss of responsibility for simple household tasks, the presence of demanding grandchildren or even the demands of the caring child for rewarding conversation and activity may be too much for the fading dement. To the child the persistent presence of a slightly drab, slow, aspontaneous yet proud parent produces a drag on the natural flow of living. Accepting responsibility for personal activities may be difficult, although probably responsive to outside support.

Of these dementing elderly people falling out of the private world of family into touch with statutory services, some will find their way to the general practitioner either because of the dementia or, more likely, because of another identified process, and others will make contact with a social services department. These professionals will formulate the identified needs in the ways they have been trained – probably. Thus the medical practitioner will review the history and examine the current state. This may result in his making a series of diagnoses among which it is said he will commonly omit the concept of dementia until its very latest stages,[44] though he may well view the patient as senile or confused. Social workers are more likely to formulate unmet needs than luxuriate on family dynamics among their elderly clients.[45] In many instances these 'primary care' agents will feel and be competent in dealing with the situation and are able to help the elderly person to maintain a supported life at home. Medicines, walking sticks, modifications to the house, nursing expertise, home help, meals on wheels, neighbourhood warden, etc. may be amongst the useful prescriptions available. At the primary care level there is a happy flexibility of response, though this varies with the interests and skills of individual practitioners and the generosity of local provision. In most areas there has been a rapid growth in the expenditure on domiciliary aids used by the elderly over the past twenty years. Not surprisingly, a household which includes a person suffering from dementia is likely to be receiving some of these services; an assessment in Newcastle in the 1960s suggested that about half the needs of demented people at home were being met by domiciliary services then available to them.[46] There are many areas now where services are of the order of double those in Newcastle of the early 1960s, and it may be that in such areas most of the help that could reasonably be expected in the homes of people suffering from dementia is being provided.

**Care in Institutions**

It is at the level where needs or problems escalate beyond the capabilities of primary care and domiciliary agencies that failings are most apparent. On the one hand, this may arise when special investigation and/or expertise is required beyond that possible in the out-patient clinic; on the other, it may be clear that what is needed is supervision of a quality and/or quantity not within the capacity of domiciliary care.

The history of hospital services for the elderly is a little difficult to disentangle. The mental hospital system evolved to provide for those who were suffering from mental disorders, with nursing skills and medical involvement superior to that of the workhouse.

The acutely ill would be managed in acute, often voluntary, hospitals with those left with chronic problems moving on to 'chronic sickness' units. Mental hospitals have always housed some elderly people, most of them suffering from mental disorders, at least at the time of admission. Yet a few are undoubtedly physically ill at first contact and others become physically dependent after a time in care. Chronic sickness hospitals housed many mentally impaired old people, particularly among the very old, and in McKeown's survey of the Birmingham Regional Board's hospitals in the 1950s there were more very elderly people (85 years or more) in need of nursing because of mental infirmity in chronic sickness hospitals than in mental hospitals.[47] Certainly most old people admitted to geriatric care are physically ill at the time, but many have mental impairments too. In those cases where the physical problem is ameliorated, the remaining mental disability alone may preclude discharge. There is no established history of transfers between mental hospital and geriatric hospitals despite this well recognised similarity in the characteristics and needs of their elderly clients. Local authority residential care has grown out of the workhouse system and a good deal of anxiety and guilt still attach to the idea of 'going into care'with the implication of freedom surrendered and an expectation of life of the lowest quality. The situation described as 'The Last Refuge' by Townsend after his meticulous and comprehensive studies of the 1950s certainly had many shortcomings.[48] A large proportion of the accommodation at that time remained in former Public Assistance buildings which housed large numbers, many very disabled, in spartan circumstances. Since then most authorities have done away with their workhouses and rely on converted mansions or purpose-built homes with around forty residents each. Thus the quality of accommodation has risen and in many respects the care offered is admirable. Yet it remains true that many residents are disabled, some being indistinguishable from the clients of geriatric and psychogeriatric hospitals even at admission,[49] and others become disabled during their stay because of the nature of the disease processes that have rendered them socially inadequate. The thought that better accommodation or other social manipulations will prevent all the ravages of old age is a forlorn hope. The only way that old people's homes could be filled with fit and lively old folk would be by rigorous exclusion of the disabled on admission and expulsion of those that become disabled after a time in residence. Thus it is that welfare homes include many residents that share the characteristics common to the long-stay patients of geriatric and psychogeriatric hospitals.[50]

These three components of residential care available to old people meet the one basic requirement that allows them to cater for people suffering from dementia: the availability of supervision every hour of the day and night. They all three contain high concentrates of dementia and none of them is very happy about this for all will see their time spent more fruitfully, more rewardingly, caring for other species of client. Psychiatric services have sought to reduce their beds and support people in the community in the chronic phases of illness. In association with their removal from mental hospitals into general hospital units they have assumed a self-image of highly skilled 'curative' potential. Such an image allows no place for the presence of old people suffering from dementia and can only be sustained when someone else provides for these people 'who do not require the skills of a [modern] psychiatrist'. The present ration of beds set aside by government for psychiatric in-patient care to elderly suffering severe dementia in England and Wales represents a freezing of the provision that practice with such a philosophy had allowed to develop by 1971.[52] Thus it is possible that further erosion of this potential haven has been prevented by this statutory directive.

Geriatric medicine has developed as a service speciality out of the chronic sickness hospitals by exposing potential clients to good clinical medicine, rehabilitation and after-care services.[53] The first generation of geriatricians has struggled hard and long with unfashionable facilities and established an image to be proud of. This includes the probability of return home after a period in hospital for the patient, and the opportunity to exercise the skills of a physician among old people for the doctor. That the impact on the patient's condition may not be quite as impressive as the escalating bed-usage figures is probably not very important, for the manner of care is important.[54] But there is a move to denigrate the skills associated with care for the chronically ill. The time of the physician can be taken up by 'treatable' problems and thus for many a geriatrician 'the service can only attain its full potential if someone else looks after those suffering from dementia'. Yet local authority homes as presently conceived cannot attend to the needs of all demented people 'in care'. Indeed the officers in charge of some complain that there are more disabled, especially confused, in homes now than was ever intended. They are right. These good women (and men) feel cheated and wish to exercise their skills in attending to the last years of more cheerful and responsive clients. Some will say it is not right that normal old people should suffer the indignity of life alongside the obviously demented. For many sound reasons: 'they should be provided for elsewhere'.

On all sides is a feeling that enough is enough and too much is sickening. What price a high-kudos assessment unit that dares to suggest residential care of some sort is required and finds itself providing just that? The ration of residential care across the hospital-local authority spectrum is now considerably less than that provided to former generations of elderly.[55] Thus in 1911, when only the fittest survived into late life and very few endured into the ninth and tenth decades, 5.3 per cent of the population over 65 years of age were in institutions of one sort of another. Among the most thought-provoking statistics that Townsend brings to our attention is the note that whilst overall institutional provision had recovered from 3.5 per cent in 1951 to 4.5 per cent in 1961 and 1966 and 4.7 per cent in 1971, the provision within mental hospitals fell progressively from 1.0 per cent in 1961 to 0.9 in 1966 and 0.8 in 1971. Thus there is within our diminished ration of residential care a progressively reduced element of specialist psychiatric provision. Indeed if current plans come to fruition, as surely they will unless the strong arguments against them are accepted by those that hold the purse strings, the contribution of mental hospitals will eventually deteriorate to 0.3-0.4 per cent elderly (this is based on the ration currently established of 0.25-0.3 per cent for dementia with a small addition for non-demented mentally ill old people). Yet there is no evidence that the number of mentally ill old people will be reduced; quite the contrary. Whilst people with non-dementing illnesses can often be helped, these illnesses do not diminish life expectation to any marked extent and it will remain necessary that sheltered accommodation of some sort be provided for them.

The number and proportion of elderly people suffering from dementia will increase markedly: using Nielsen's figures,[56] the prevalence of dementia rises from 4.2 per cent (none severe) at 65-69 years through 26.0 per cent (2.2 severe) at 75-79 years to 60 per cent (17.8 severe) in the 85+ age group. These, together with estimates of change within the old age population which include increasing salience of very old people, give a roughly calculated estimate that whilst the total population of pensioners will have increased by 150 per cent in the second half of this century, the number suffering from dementia will have increased 175 per cent and the severely demented by 200 per cent. The impact of this spectacular increase will be magnified even further; for we have seen that it is just this group of dements – those living alone after a lifetime with others – who cannot be successfully maintained at home even with the provision of skilled day hospital support in addition to other forms of domiciliary care.[57]

Present patterns of institutional care suggest that very elderly dements are usually successfully managed in welfare homes. Yet the essence of these establishments as a 'non-hospital' environment is that they include a fair percentage of relatively able folk. Even if extra care is provided in terms of hours and specialist skills of nurses, occupational therapists and physiotherapists, it would seem necessary that for every severely disabled resident there should be about four less disabled. Thus providing institutional care for these extra demented old people in welfare homes would require something like five new beds for every bed currently available to demented people in mental hospitals: this would probably produce the best-balanced and highest quality of care for elderly dements and it may be that it will be achieved.

In the interim a relatively simple manipulation would produce a viable, if less than ideal, alternative, by maintaining the number of mental hospital beds currently available to the elderly and redistributing them as the needs arise so that most become used by the demented.

## Psychogeriatric Services

Interest in the provision of services to mentally ill old people was founded in Duncan MacMillan's service in Nottingham. Such enterprises have gained recognition and respect and are now attracting recruits in reasonable number and quality. Much of the recent success must be attributed to the efforts of pioneers such as R.A. Robinson, Brice Pitt, Klaus Bergmann, Tony Whitehead and Tom Arie for their example and attractive merchandising of the new subspeciality. All have

**Figure 5.1: Changing Expectations of Demented Elderly Seeking Residential Care, 1911-2011**

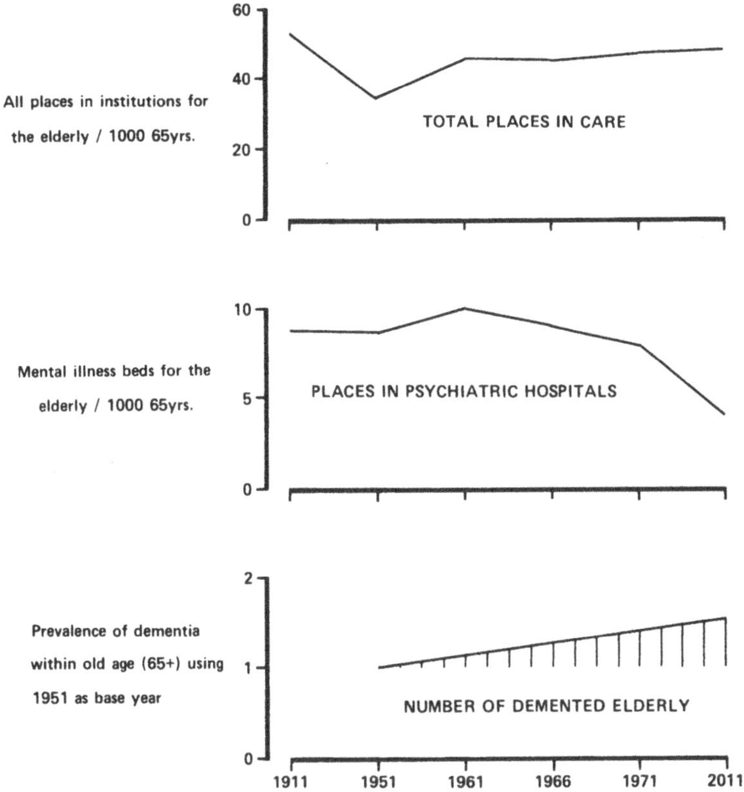


warned against preoccupation with glamorous assessment units and rightly stressed the satisfaction associated with ultimate responsibility for continuing care. Most of the early services have been hewn out of the massive bed numbers available in mental hospitals and have produced active, lively responses to community needs by providing domiciliary assessment, day hospital support, supervision at home through social workers and community nurses as well as assessment and treatment on an out-patient, day-patient or in-patient basis. It has been usual for these services to confine their efforts to providing for people falling ill in old age[58] and at least half the mentally ill elderly in hospital – the so-called 'graduates' – have remained in the care of general psychiatrists. Despite well presented suggestions that 'psychogeriatricians' should widen their interests to include the 'graduates',[59] the massive work-load involved with current job descriptions have made the proposition unacceptable to most. Yet we are moving towards a time when generations of mentally ill people will graduate into old age having been supported outside hospital by community care and medication. The pressures on psychogeriatric services to accept responsibility for these people, or at least make sure adequate provision is available, will grow and begin to compete for attention and resources with the doubled case-load of dementia. With energetic and interested management many will be maintained with little or no recourse to hospital beds – but the new subspeciality of 'Psychiatry of Old Age' must make a statement about its resource requirements to meet the predictable needs of its present and future clients. The arguments enumerated in current policy[51] do not hold up to the severe examination which derives from epidemiological trends. Certainly it would seem that until adequate alternative accommodation is made available, we should ensure that mental illness hospital provision for the elderly is not reduced below its present ration, i.e., 8 beds for every 1,000 aged 65 years and more. This has the advantage of making it clear that the needs of the elderly led by those suffering dementia require a redistribution of psychiatric manpower even greater than that currently envisaged by the Royal College of Psychiatrists.[60] It is unlikely that this reasonable ploy will be greeted with rapture, but it would provide a chance that this country's other caring services are not overwhelmed by a sea of elderly dements. The only other alternative is to deny people with dementia access to available caring establishments and leave them and their families to suffer the ravages of the disease.

It is scarcely believable that such an old-fashioned illness must inevitably cause such chaos and suffering in this year and the years to come. A good deal of suffering can be diminished if society will bring itself to direct resources to those modes of care that are known to be successful. Yet it remains doubtful whether we have the maturity to accept such a course in preference to appearing to do the impossible by tolerating statistics that fail to reflect real needs,[61] or finding solace in false philosophy that makes virtue of neglect.[62]

## References

1. Hunt, A. (1978) *The Elderly at Home*, HMSO, London
2. Clarke, M. *et al.* (1979) *Health Trends, 1,* 11, 17
3. de Beauvoir, S. (1977) *Old Age*, Penguin, Harmondsworth, Middlesex
4. Post, F. (1965) *The Clinical Psychiatry of Late Life*, Pergamon Press, Oxford

5. Roth, M., and Morrissey, J.D. (1952) *Journal of Mental Science, 98*, 66
6. Post, F. (1962) *The Signifcance of Affective Symptoms in Old Age*, Oxford University Press, London
7. Kay, D.W.K. (1959) *Proc. Royal Society of Medicine, 52*, 791
8. Post, F. (1966) *Persistent Persecutory States of the Elderly*, Pergamon Press, Oxford
9. Kay, D.W.K., Beamish, P., and Roth, M. (1964) *British Journal of Psychiatry, 110*, 146
10. Parsons, P.L. (1965) *British Journal of Preventive and Social Medicine, 19*, 43
11. Bremer, J. (1951) 'A Social Psychiatric Investigation of a Small Community in Northern Norway', *Acta Psychiatrica Scandinavica*, Suppl. 62
12. Gruenberg, E.M. (1961) *A Mental Health Survey of Older People*, State Hospitals Press, New York
13. Bergmann, K. (1971) 'The Neuroses of Old Age' in D.W.K. Kay and A. Walk (eds.), *Recent Developments in Psychogeriatrics*, Headley Bros., Ashford, Kent
14. McKechnie, A. (1978) MD thesis, University of Aberdeen
15. Lishman, W.A. (1978) *Organic Psychiatry*, Blackwell Scientific Publications, Oxford
16. Jolley, D.J., and Arie, T. (1980) *Health Trends, 12*, 1
17. Arie, T. (1973) *British Medical Journal, 3*, 540 and 602
18. Hachinski, V.C., Lassen, N.A., and Marshall, J. (1974) *Lancet, 2*, 207
19. Roth, M. (1955) *Journal of Mental Science, 101*, 281
20. Kay, D.W.K. (1962) *Acta Psychiatrica Scandinavica, 28*, 249
21. MacDonald, C. (1969) *British Journal of Psychiatry, 115*, 267
22. Fisk, J. (1979) M. Phil. thesis, University of Edinburgh
23. Isaacs, B. (1972) *The Survival of the Unfittest*, Routledge and Kegan Paul, London
24. Godber, C. (1977) in R. Glasscote, J.E. Gudeman and D. Miles (edn.), *Creative Mental Health Services for the Elderly* Joint Information Services of American Psychiatric Association and Mental Health Association, *Washington, DC*
25. Gruenberg, E.M. (1978) *Advances in Neurology, 19*, 437
26. Larssen, T., Sjogren, T., and Jacobsen, G. (1963) *Acta Psychiatrica Scandinavica*, Suppl. 167
27. Kay, D.W.K., Beamish, P., and Roth, M. (1964) *British Journal of Psychiatry, 110*, 668
28. Isaacs, B., and Neville, Y. (1976) *British Journal of Preventive and Social Medicine, 30*, 79
29. Jefferys, M. (1978) 'The Elderly in Society' in J.C. Brocklehurst (ed.), *Textbook of Geriatric Medicine and Gerontology*, Churchill-Livingstone, Edinburgh
30. Slater, E., and Cowie, V. (1971) *The Genetics of Mental Disorders*, Oxford University Press, London
31. Nielsen, J. (1968) *British Journal of Psychiatry, 114*, 303
32. Olsen, M.I., and Shaw, G.M. (1969) *Brain, 92*, 147
33. Levy, R., Isaacs, A., and Hawks, G. (1970) *Psychological Medicine, 1*, 40
34. Corsellis, J.A.N. (1962) *Mental Illness and the Ageing Brain*, Oxford University Press, London
35. Tomlinson, B.E., Blessed, G., and Roth, M. (1970) *Journal of Neurological Sciences, 11*, 205
36. Bowen, D.M., and Davison, A.N. (1978) in B. Isaacs, *Recent Advances in Geriatric Medicine*, Churchill-Livingstone, Edinburgh
37. Perry, E. *et al.* (1978) *British Medical Journal; 2*, 1457

38. Mann, D.M.A., Yates, P.O., and Barton, C.M. (1977) *Journal of Neurology, Neurosurgery and Psychiatry, 40*, 299
39. Sutton, R.N.P., and Lord, A. (1978) 'Slow Viruses and Neurological Diseases' in J.D. Williams (ed.), *Modern Topics in Infection*, Heinemann Medical Books, London
40. Marshall, J. (1973) *British Journal of Hospital Medicine, 10*, 240
41. Wollner, L., McCarthy, S.T., Soper, N.D.W., and Macy, D.J. (1979) *British Medical Journal, 1,* 1117
42. *British Medical Journal* (1979), editorial, *2*, 511
43. Woods, R.T., and Britton, P.G. (1977) *Age and Ageing, 6*, 104
44. Williamson, J. Stokoe, I.H., Gray, S., Fisher, M., Smith, A., McGhee, A., and Stevenson, E. (1964) *Lancet, 1*, 117
45. Goldberg, E.M. *et al.* (1977) *British Journal of Social Work, 7*, 3, 258
46. Foster, E.M., Kay, D.W.K., and Bergmann, K. (1976) *Age and Ageing, 5*, 245
47. McKeown, T., Mackintosh, J., and Lowe, C.R. (1961) *Lancet, 1,* 818
48. Townsend, P. (1962) *The Last Refuge*, Routledge and Kegan Paul, London
49. Smith, R.G., and Lowther, C.P. (1976) *Age and Ageing, 5*, 176
50. Wilkin, D., Jolley, D.J. (1978) *Nursing Times*, Occasional Paper, *74*, 117, 124
51. DHSS (1972) *Services for Mental Illness Related to Old Age*, HM (72) 71, HMSO, London
52. Jolley, D.J. (1977) *British Medical Journal, 1*, 1335
53. Williamson, J.(1979) *Age and Ageing, 8*, 144
54. Nisbett, N.H. (1970) *Lancet, 1*, 133
55. The Disability Alliance (1979) *The Government's Failure to Plan for Disablement in Old Age* (principal author Peter Townsend)
56. Neilsen, J. (1962) *Acta Psychiatrica Scandinavica, 38*, 307
57. Bergmann, K., Foster, E.M., Justice, A.W., and Matthews, V. (1978) *British Journal of Psychiatry, 132*, 44
58. Jolley, D.J. and Arie, T. (1978) *British Journal of Psychiatry, 132*, 1
59. McDonald, C. (1979) *Geriatric Medicine, 9*, 6, 53
60. Royal College of Psychiatrists (1975), *British Journal of Psychiatry*, News and Notes, July, 3
61. Arie, T. (1973) 'Psychiatric Needs of the Elderly' in *Needs of the Elderly for Health and Welfare Services*, Exeter University Press, Exeter
61. Opit, M. (1977) *British Medical Journal, 1*, 30

# 6 AFFECTIVE ILLNESSES

Felix Post

## Introduction

Affective illnesses in old age are characterised by the same abnormalities of mood as those encountered in younger people: sadness or a lowering of affective state down to emptiness and detachment; anxiety rising to panic states: and euphoric elation sometimes increasing to excitement. In many patients various mixtures of these pathological mood-states may be encountered. The altered affect is usually well described by the patient, unless it is very severe and inhibits communication, or the patient is poorly verbally endowed. In addition, the affective disturbance is experienced and communicated by psychomotor behaviour: facial expression, gesturing and general body motility. The specifically human psychomotor function of speech is always affected in mood disorders: with sadness and emotional emptiness it is slowed, diminished or even almost extinguished; in anxiety, speech tends to become speeded up and excessive in quantity, but repetitive and importuning in content; with elation and excitement, speech will become not only excessive, but disorganised, sometimes beyond the limits of comprehensibility. The patient's spoken and written productions reveal that the mood disorder has to a varying extent affected his thoughts about himself and the world around him. Sadness is associated with lowering of self-esteem and decreased interest in the surroundings; in severe cases firm beliefs of the patient's wickedness in past and present are expressed; related to this the contents of the body are experienced as bad. With anxiety, self-worth or evaluation of the past are less affected, but fears are experienced concerning disease and other future threats to life and security. In milder cases these fears are recognised as imaginary, but cannot be banished altogether. In elated states, the patient shows to a pathological degree over-valuations of his personality, past achievements and future prospects. In all but the mildest affective illnesses, sleep, appetite, body weight regulation and a number of other so-called vital functons are to a varying extent disordered.

In this chapter, I shall first describe in more detail the pictures presented by affective disorders in late life; I shall next discuss briefly their treatment, and more fully their outcome in relation to modern therapies; finally, I shall be speculating on their causation.

## Depressive Illnesses

The first appearance of depressive illnesses in real old age, i.e. after 75, severe enough to require medical or psychiatric consultations, is unusual. On the other hand, large numbers of patients with affective illnesses who are in their seventies or eighties are seen in psychiatric out-patient or in-patient facilities. Most of them, however, will be suffering from recurrences of depressions since an earlier age. In technical terms, there is thus a lower incidence but a high prevalence of affective disorders during old age. Affective illnesses appear for the first time with increasing frequency from adolescence on right through adult life, but the more severe forms have their greatest incidence between the ages of 40 and 65. At that age, incidence declines, but occasionally a first attack may occur in the late eighties, or even during the tenth decade of life. Milder depressions reach their highest incidence between 40 and 50.[1,2]

On the other hand, mood disorders which take the form of subjective complaints, and which rarely become known to any doctor, are very frequent in the elderly: in up to 40 per cent of a sample of American community subjects volunteering for a research project[3] (though rather less frequently in those with meaningful occupations and interests); in only 5 per cent of a sample of Scottish community residents, but in 14 per cent of those attending a geriatric clinic:[4] in 32 per cent of a series coming to the notice of local authority services.[5] Hardly any of these 'complaint depressives' make suicidal attempts, let alone succeed in killing themselves.

Attempted suicide among the elderly is much less common than in younger persons, but completed suicide rates increase, especially in the case of men, right into old age, and moreover they tend to be related to clinical depressions, occasionally in a setting of early cerebral decline.[6,7]

Regardless of the age at which the first attack had occurred, depressives admitted to psychiatric hospitals present with three fairly well differentiated types of clinical picture.[8]

First of all, there are severely psychotic depressives who communicate clearly by their general bearing a severe mood of sadness, hopelessness and, usually in this age group, dread and fear. In these severe affective disturbances there is seen very marked slowing or agitation, usually both in quick succession. Most of these patients voice delusional ideas concerning physical ill health, poverty, guilt or self-depreciation; some may feel that they are persecuted or even legally prosecuted for imagined misdeeds. They may believe that bad smells emanate from them; hypochondriacal delusions and psychotic depersonalisation may take on a bizarre and nihilistic form, and accusations may assume the character of pseudo-hallucinatory voices. Some practically mute patients are obviously so severely ill that melancholic disorders of experiencing and thought content can only be surmised as being present but may not be demonstrable. Dementia may be suspected, and in these very ill patients this condition cannot be immediately excluded.

Next, there are psychotic depressives with any of the above psychopathological phenomena, but only one of two kinds tend to be present at the same time. Paranoid symptoms, not only of a clearly guilt-ridden kind, are especially common in this group, and hypochondriacal delusions are perhaps less common in this group of depressives than abnormal ideas concerning self-worth. The affect, however, seems empty and flat rather than overtly depressed or panic-stricken: it may be surly and hostile, and the descriptive term of 'aversion-depression' comes to mind. These patients are likely to be misdiagnosed as so-called senile paraphrenics by the uninitiated.

Third, there are neurotic depressives, who preserve at most times the capacity to see that their fears and thoughts are likely to be due to their emotional state: they apprehend that they might have some abdominal obstruction, but are for a time reassured by negative physical examinations. They realise that their self-depreciatory attitude may be unjustified. In addition, these patients frequently exhibit phobias (especially of going out or of staying indoors on their own) or, more rarely, obsessive-compulsive phenomena. Histrionic rather than fully fledged hysterical features are also fairly frequent. Depression in this group of patients is not very strongly communicated to the doctor, but anxiety is more obvious. Importantly, there are some patients who complain of hypochondriacal sensations and fears, various neurotic problems, but who do not appear even to the trained observed to be either depressed or anxious. Anxiety is not, as in younger people, experienced and communicated in terms of tremor, dilated pupils, sweating or palpitations, but rather as general restlessness and unpleasant body sensations, especially fluttering feelings in the abdomen. Some of these patients do not respond to family doctor or out-patient treatment and require admission to hospital because they become too disturbing to their relatives on account of continuous complaints. Also they sometimes neglect themselves and lose weight to a similar extent as patients exhibiting psychotic clinical pictures.

It is not known whether any one of these three sub-types is more prone to suicidal behaviour than the others. Accounts of the way in which these three types of depression had taken hold of individual patients do not suggest that neurotic depression represents the early and initial stage of psychotic depression. Also, all three described types of depressions represent overlapping symptom clusters rather than sharply distinguished clinical states. There is one exception: a strong impression exists that, during the further course taken by those severe psychotics who fail to respond to treatment by complete or considerable remission of symptoms these patients may lose a good deal of severe sadness and distress with which one easily feels empathy, and come to approach the state of deluded, but relatively affectless, psychotics.

Almost certainly, as in the case of younger patients, neurotic depressive pictures are far more common than psychotic forms. Many neurotic depressives do not come to be counted at all, either because they do not see their doctors, or more likely because their doctors treat them for their somatic complaints alone. Increasing numbers are now recognised as depressives by their family doctors, but many of them never refer any old people to psychiatrists. So, the elderly neurotic depressives ultimately seen by psychiatrists after unsuccessful general practitioner treatment or possibly after suicidal attempts, are likely to be quite atypical of the general run of elderly neurotic depressives. By contrast, psychotic depressives almost always come into psychiatric care sooner or later.

As far as management and treatment are concerned, I have been unimpressed by the value of any therapies which do not attack the mood disorder at central nervous system level. Attention to general health, including the effective treatment of significant and possibly precipitating physical conditions, seems to have little effect on the depression. On the psychological side, 'working through' a bereavement reaction does not seem to affect the depressive state once it has become established. I even recall vividly a patient with previous depressions in whom my attempts at working through her husband's pending death singularly failed to prevent a further attack! Family relations of neurotic depressives often tend to be problematical, but again attention to these aspects does not ease the patient's depression. Psycho- and socio-therapeutic activities are all the same useful, even essential, because they seem to facilitate the effect of drug therapy by increasing compliance with antidepressant regimes, and also by making agreement to undergo electroconvulsive therapy, if that becomes indicated, more likely. In the many instances where treatment has been unsuccessful, or only partially successful, social casework and supportive psychotherapy may make the continuing state of mental ill health or invalidism more tolerable to both patient and family. However, before turning in more detail to the management of depression, we have to draw attention to a second form of affective disorder of the elderly, the importance of which may have been underestimated in the past.

**Manic Conditions**

Among the case records of all patients over the age of 60 admitted to the in-patient facilities of the Bethlem Royal and Maudsley hospitals over a ten-year period, there were 67 in whom diagnosis of either manic or manic-depressive illness could be substantiated.[9] The number of depressives over 60 passing during the same period through the wards of these hospitals was not ascertained, but in one earlier study[8] it had been found that 17 among the 92 elderly depressives investigated had at one time or other exhibited manic states. Among the 67 patients of the more recent investigation,[9] manic symptoms had occurred for the first time before the age of 40 in only 6 cases, and only 5 patients suffered manic attacks for the first time in life after the age of 69. The average age at first manic attack was 58.9 years. The female over male preponderance was 2.7:1, i.e. higher than has been found to be the case in elderly depressives (1.7:1), but nothing like as high as in so-called late paraphrenics. In two-thirds of cases the first mental breakdown had been depressive, and in the remainder either purely manic or mixed manic-depressive. Up to 47 years were found to have passed between the first depression and the first manic attack, though the average 'latency period' amounted to only 10 years. In just over half, three or more depressive attacks were counted before the onset of mania, indicating how unrealiable and premature the categorisation of a patient as suffering from a uni-polar depression will be when it is made before old age is reached.

Regarding the clinical picture of mania in the elderly, I used to accept previous views that ageing had an important pathoplastic influence: there was said to be only rarely in elderly manics infectious elation, but more often a surly and aggressive mood. Talk was said to be less often indicative of a rapid, but more likely of a slow, flight of ideas; moreover, senile anecdotalism and circumstantiality would often colour speech productions. Also, it was held that pure manic states hardly ever occurred in the elderly so that some depressive colouring was always in evidence. Now I am not so sure, as classical flights of ideas are not really all that frequent in younger manics, in whom depressive affects are also almost always in evidence to the discerning clinician. The frequency of depressive admixtures, even in manic children and adolescents, has been pointed out recently.[10] The treatment of elderly manics with tranquillisers and lithium salts does not differ from that of younger patients.

## Outcome in Relation to Modern Therapy

Most depressives, whatever their age, are treated successfully by family doctors, general physicians and, in the case of the elderly, by geriatricians. The efficacy of antidepressant drugs in depressives belonging to the older age groups does not seem to have been specifically studied, nor have there been any reports of elderly depressives treated in psychiatric out-patient clinics. Treatment and its outcome in nearly 100 depressives over the age of 60 during their in-patient stay and during the first three years after discharge were scrutinised a few years ago,[8] and a comparison with the treatment and outcome of an equally large but earlier sample of in-patients was undertaken.

It emerged that among the patients admitted around 1950 only 15 per cent had received any treatment prior to admission, while around 1966 treatment (mainly with antidepressants, which had of course not yet been introduced in the early 1950s) had been given without much benefit to 61 per cent of depressives before they had to be admitted. In other words, we are now treating as psychiatric in-patients, and probably also as out-patients, a higher proportion of persons with the more resistant kinds of illness, and this very likely holds with special force in the case of the neurotic forms of the disorder. So anything one can say about treatment and prognosis of hospitalised elderly depressives cannot be applied without further thought to elderly depressives remaining in the community: most of the more readily treatable and less ill patients are now creamed off by family doctors and out-patient facilities, and it is therefore not really surprising that the therapeutic results achieved with hospital cases in 1950 turned out to have been not significantly better than those obtained in 1966. By then initial hospital stay had certainly been shortened, but re-admission rates had increased, and more seriously, there were 10 as against only 4 suicide attempts in the later sample during a much shorter follow-up period. Three as against only one patient of the earlier series succeeded in killing themselves.

During their index illness, just under half of patients of the 1966 sample received ECT either soon after admission or after tricyclic drugs had failed. The proportion of patients receiving ECT around 1950 was only insignificantly higher: just over half. A third of the later sample remitted on tricyclics alone, and about a fifth had been given monoamine oxidase inhibitors. One patient in each sample had psychosurgery, which is nowadays only rarely recommended. As we shall see presently, there is no dearth of patients failing to respond to non-invasive types of therapy, and who might perhaps benefit from psychosurgery. But chronic and intractable depressives in our age group also tend to be physically frail and possibly cerebrally impaired, and thus not suitable for brain surgery. In a large proportion of patients suitable for psychosurgery, they or their relatives withhold informed consent in the present climate of public opinon. The few apparently irretrievably ill patients who recently had operations have done as well as early results of modified leucotomies in elderly patients had indicated.

Turning to the results achieved in hospital patients by the various forms of treatment, only about a quarter remained completely well over the subsequent three years, and just over a third suffered further attacks, but made good remissions in between. On the other hand, a quarter did not remit completely and continued to suffer from what one might call depressive invalidism, as well as from further exacerbations, in most cases. Just over a tenth of patients remained in states of chronic and unremitting depression. It has recently been pointed out [11,12] that complete restitution to previous mental health is not all that frequently achieved in younger depressives either, and that, as so often, the textbooks have been wrong in claiming complete remissions and good adjustment in between attacks of affective illness. In accordance with the unfavourable long-term course pursued by most of our patients, treatment could be lastingly stopped in only 25 per cent. The remainder required continuously or intermittently further antidepressant measures, including ECT in nearly 20 per cent. Active, as against expectant, social work made little difference to long-term outcome, except perhaps for bringing old people earlier into repeated treatment.

Since these experiences were gathered, there have been two important developments, neither of which has, however, been scientifically checked specifically for elderly depressives. The first is the introduction of lithium therapy which, as was stated earlier, together with the use of major tranquillisers, had been found just as effective in elderly manics as in younger ones. In addition, in recent years it has been our practice to place on lithium maintenance therapy any depressives who were physically fit for it, and who had suffered recently more than one depressive attack annually. My strong impression is that no patient whose plasma lithium levels remained within the therapeutic range suffered serious recurrences, but that attempts at discontinuing maintenance therapy sooner rather than later led to serious recurrences in every instance.

The other recent development concerns the monitoring of blood levels of antidepressant drugs. There are still differences of opinion among the experts, but impressionistically it certainly has been my experience that both too low and too high blood levels of antidepressant drugs are attended by therapeutic failure, which can often be reversed by adjustment of dosage. It has become my practice to ask for drug levels if after a fortnight or so during which daily dosages had been built up to the equivalent of, say, amitripyline 150 mgs no worthwhile clinical improvement had occurred. The need to avoid unecessarily high doses in old people requires no emphasis.

Finally, one may ask whether there are any features which would allow one to predict long-term outcome in the presence of effective therapy: the answer is no, as far as the individual patient is concerned. Complete remission of the index illness is a good sign, but this is difficult to determine now when so many patients leave hospital while still on antidepressants. On the whole, patients whose recurrent illnesses commenced early in life do better than those with what used to be called involutional and senile depressions. Extraverted personalities do best. Age over 70 and physical debilities associated with old age are related to a poorer prognosis. Though patients with proved cerebral pathology, for example depressed stroke patients, quite often respond well to therapy directed towards their mood disorder, their relapse rate is high. When paranoid symptomatology approaches the kind which by expert consensus would be regarded as schizophrenic, i.e. in schizoaffective cases, outlook is poor.[2]

### Some Speculations Concerning Causation

Speculations concerning aetiology are obviously of general and theoretical interest. If we knew more precisely how it sometimes goes wrong, we might learn a lot about how the human mind ticks! From a medical practical point of view, immeasurable benefits would accrue to patients if we had firm knowledge of the ways in which their breakdowns had been caused. Keeping in mind the complexity of the human mind and of the milieu in which it operates, simple and single causes of its derangement are unlikely to be discovered. But if only one could unravel the many factors operating in psychic illnesses, no doubt some of them might prove remediable.

In the case of the more severe affective disorders, it has long been known that they have a constitutional basis: depressive psychoses tend to run in families, victims of the disorder tend to exhibit certain types of body build and, even more clearly demonstrable, certain types of personality structure. Probably little can be done to change these constitutional predispositions to affective illness, though some successes have been claimed for psychoanalytical treatment in preventing or ameliorating recurrent affective psychoses by modifying personality.

Equally strong evidence has been assembled for the aetiological importance of environmental stresses. Most of it is so well established that there is no need to refer to specific items in the literature, for example the undue frequency of the loss during childhood of a parent in persons developing depressive illnesses in adult life. The impact of parental attitudes is less well documented, but would obviously hold greater prophylactic possibilities. More recently, it has become almost axiomatic that attacks of affective illness follow upon disruptive life events far more frequently than could be explained by chance coincidence. At the same time, research has reminded us that environmental stresses cannot possibly be the sole causes of depression: in a control population experiencing similar recent events as a group of patients with precipitated depressions, only 9 per cent developed the disorder: so, in scientific jargon, 'the greater part of the variance must be explained by something else'.[13] This argument is especially cogent for the psychiatrist with special interest in the aged, who if it were not for this 'something else' would expect practically every old person eventually to succumb with a depressive illness to the severe stresses to which elderly people are invariably exposed: all the kinds of losses known to precipitate depression at all ages, like bereavement, removal of close associates, loss of self-esteem after retirement, loss of the accustomed home, to name only a few, are sooner or later experienced by all ageing persons.

Finally, at a much more practical level, it would be of great benefit to the patient if the type of his affective illness could be used as an indicator for a specific kind of therapy. I indicated earlier in this chapter that it was fairly easy to divide elderly depressives into three descriptive types: severely psychotic, moderately psychotic and neurotic depressives. It might be assumed that electroconvulsive therapy would be more effective in psychotic than in predominantly neurotic patients, who might be expected to respond better to antidepressant drugs without any need to resort to ECT. Certainly, more psychotics than neurotics are as a first choice treated with ECT, which in situations of considerable urgency tends to produce beneficial results much earlier. However, it was discovered that, in the long run, remission as indicated by discharge from hospital was achieved by ECT only insignificantly more frequently than through the use of pharmacological agents, regardless of whether the patient had suffered from a psychotic or a neurotic depression.[8] From a theoretical angle, it might be expected that in comparison with neurotic depressives, psychotic depressives, who are also often called 'endogenous depressives', would show stronger constitutional defects and fewer life events preceding their illnesses.

However, against expectation, none of these suggested associations could be confirmed at a statistically acceptable level. To give an example, psychotics with a slightly stronger family history of depression registered precipitation by life events more frequently than neurotic depressives as a group! The symptomatology of a depressive illness is almost certainly profoundly influenced by the previous personality. In comparing psychotic with neurotic depressives, the latter had suffered from independently attested neurotic personality problems highly significantly more often than the psychotics.[8] Taking into account not only symptomatology, but also heredity, background and life experiences, it proved impossible to allocate elderly depressives sufficiently ill to enter hospital to any separate diagnostic category like 'endogenous' or 'reactive'.[2,8]

It has now been widely recognised[14] that in the present state of our ignorance, choice of therapy should not be influenced by types of symptomatology or aetiological factors, and that our efforts should simply be limited to remedying the affective disturbance. The form which a depressive illness takes will of course influence our management: it shows common sense to arrange early admission of the psychotic, but to attempt ambulant treatment with drugs of the neurotic depressive.

Continuing our speculations along entirely theoretical lines, research into affective disorders of late life has been limited almost entirely to the depressive variety, on account of the relative rarity of manic pictures. We saw earlier that elderly depressives encountered in psychiatric practice are either patients who had been suffering recurrent affective breakdowns since a younger age, or persons developing depressive tendencies only late in life. By comparing these two types of depressives attempts have been made to unravel aetiological factors of depression specifically operating only in late life.

Regarding constitutional factors, almost all workers have found that, in comparison with life-long depressives, hereditary genetic factors were much less in evidence in cases of late onset.[15] Also, by and large, late life depressives have been found to possess tougher personalities than those with early onset illnesses.[16] It seemed natural and commonsensical to conclude that for these reasons an accumulation of adverse life events in old age, especially of various kinds of losses, might be the main aetiological factor in late onset depressions. However, this supposition could not be confirmed: I applied stringent criteria for life events in the sense of their having taken place no more than one year before onset of depression, of having been of an incisive character, like loss or threatened loss of persons, sudden and threatening physical illness, abrupt loss of status, etc., and had been reported not just by the patient but also been obtained from other sources. It was discovered that factors of this sort had been found to have played a role in some 75 per cent of all elderly depressives, a figure very similar to that given for younger patients. Precipitating factors were, however, found no more frequently in elderly depressives with late onset than in those who had suffered recurrent attacks from an earlier age.[8,16]

Furthermore, losses and stresses of the kind just mentioned affect almost all ageing people, and while it is true that some 25 per cent of a volunteer sample in the above-quoted study[3] reported brief depressive episodes, only 1-2 per cent of old people ever develop persistent clinical depressions. None of the 25 per cent of volunteers with depressive moods[3] required psychiatric treatment during the subsequent observation period, demonstrating that an episode of unhappiness is not a mild form of a depressive illness. Why some constitutionally stable people fell depressively ill for the first time in late life during old age, and why recurrent depressives tend to have more frequent recurrences as they grow older have proved to be interesting research questions, and have been explored with a number of observations as starting-points.

Elderly depressives, especially when originally not too well endowed intellectually, and when suffering from the more psychotic types of symptoms, quite often do badly on some measures of memory and learning, while remaining sufficiently co-operative to perform at expected levels on many other tasks. It had been shown previously that this type of impairment does not affect prognosis, and that following treatment it improves in parallel with the depression. This 'pseudo-dementia' is clinically obvious in some 16 per cent of cases, but can be demonstrated in a far larger proportion, not perhaps clinically, but psychometrically.[17] The suggestion that the temporary impairment may indicate some underlying cerebral impairment, especially perhaps of the arousal systems due to age, and that this impairment may facilitate both first and further attacks of recurring depressions in late life, has been investigated. This possibility could neither be excluded[17] nor could it be more than weakly supported.[18] In any case, the memory and learning impairment found in elderly depressives has been shown to be qualitatively different from that seen in the dementias of old age.[19,20] Another observation has been recorded: that there is with rising age an increase in monoamine oxidase concentration in the brain.[21] Plausibly, this may explain a first occurrence in late life of depression, as well as the longer duration and propensity to more frequent recurrences at that time of life. Finally, on a number of anxiety and depression scales, normal old persons have been shown to obtain higher scores than younger, non-psychiatric subjects.[22]

In a recent, so far unconfirmed, study[23] minor forms of disorientation and memory defects were discovered in elderly depressives distinguished by a later onset, greater age and less favourable outcome. These authors confirmed that, as in elderly depressives as a group, the affective disorder did not represent an early stage of senile or arteriosclerotic dementia; and as I had done earlier,[24] they postulated that in late life the occcurrence and frequent recurrence of depressions might be facilitated by some more subtle age changes in the central nervous and neuro-endocrine systems. Further support for this hypothesis has come recently from a number of findings: late life depressives as a group scored even after recovery slightly lower on an intelligence test than normal controls. Elderly depressives also continued to show an abnormality of auditorily evoked cortical responses similar to but less marked than that discovered in senile dements.[25] Finally, in a sample of elderly psychiatric patients submitted to the newly introduced technique of computed tomography (EMI Scanner), 8 of 9 late onset depressives registered degrees of cerebral atrophy, which were similar to those found in elderly dements.[26]

## Some Concluding Thoughts

Affective disorders of the elderly nowadays are eminently treatable conditions. In a mild form they have a very frequent occurrence, but it seems likely that the mild depressives often go unrecognised and untreated because hypochondriacal complaints and excessive preoccupations with real physical disabilities tend to mask the underlying depression of mood, interest and zest for life and activity.

As in the case of younger persons, once an affective breakdown has occurred it seems almost always to be followed by a personality change, and in the case of the elderly also by further frequent attacks of the mood disorder. For this reason, any elderly person who has suffered a breakdown should remain under some form of supervision, and may need drug maintenance or repeated courses of treatment. In spite of these measures, patients suffering from progressive physical disease, and especially from cerebral deterioration, are likely to remain psychiatric invalids.

Affective illnesses remain an enigma. It has been shown that to blame the often unfortunate situation of the aged for their frequency in late life is tempting but inadequate. It has been suggested that, as in younger persons, biological factors are more important than environmental ones, though their impact may determine the actual moment at which breakdowns first occur.

Any attempt to explain why the period of life during which ageing gains momentum should also be the one during which there is a marked increase of the incidence and prevalence of affective illnesses should be based on an understanding of the mechanisms operating in their genesis. Some relevant but unconfirmed experimental evidence as well as some theoretical speculations have been summarised, and I am tempted to suggest a hypothesis for the origin of affective disorders in general, and for their increased prevalence and incidence in late life along the following lines.

It is suggested that the perception and impact of a variety of life events may trigger much increased activity of those deep cerebral structures which subserve both the psychic (emotional turmoil) and the physiological (enhanced psycho-motor activity) manifestations of what is called affect. This translation of psychic perception into physiological changes in central nervous and neuro-endocrine functioning and back into a subjective psychological 'feeling state' incidentally demonstrates that traditional views postulating the existence of a mind-brain barrier could now be abandoned (no less)! In order to trace the development of a psychiatric illness out of environmentally induced emotional turmoil, it is suggested that the increased activity of deep cerebral structures is experienced as anxiety and manifests itself physically as agitation. If sufficiently severe and prolonged, the bombardment with signals from deeper central structures of the limbic arousal system and possibly also of the cerebral cortex may result in Pavlovian paradoxical inhibition, leading to clinical depression, slowing and lowering of certain aspects of memory functioning. As people grow older, the occurrence of this inhibition might become increasingly facilitated by a base-line reduction of the activity of the relevant parts of the nervous and neuro-endocrine systems. This base-line reduction in the level of activity should be conceptualised as due to molecular rather than coarse structural age changes. Once therapeutic intervention in the ageing process itself becomes a reality, this may also prevent or ameliorate the age-related increased proneness to affective disorders.

## References


1. Gurland, B.J. (1976) 'The Comparative Frequency of Depression in Various Adult Age Groups', *Journal of Gerontology, 31*, 283-92
2. Post, F. (1974) 'Diagnosis of Depression in Geriatric Patients and Treatment Modalities Appropriate for the Population' in D.M. Gallant and G.D. Simpson (eds.), *Depression*, Spectrum Publications, New York
3. Gianturco, D.T., and Busse, E.W. (1978) 'Psychiatric Problems Encountered During a Longterm Study of Normal Ageing Volunteers' in A.D. Isaacs and F. Post, *Studies in Geriatric Psychiatry*, John Wiley, Chichester
4. Williamson, J. (1978) 'Depression in the Elderly', *Age and Ageing, 7* (Supp), 35-40
5. Goldberg, E.M. (1970) *Helping the Aged: a Field Experiment in Social Work*, Allen and Unwin, London
6. Barraclough, B.M. (1971) 'Suicide in the Elderly' in D.W.K. Kay and A. Walk (eds.), *Recent Developments in Psychogeriatrics*, British Journal of Psychiatry Spec. Pub. No. 6
7. Shulman, K. (1978) 'Suicide and Parasuicide in Old Age: a Review', *Age and Ageing, 7*, 201-9
8. Post, F. (1972) 'The Management and Nature of Depressive Illness in Late Life: a Follow-through Study', *British Journal of Psychiatry, 121*, 393-404
9. Shulman, K. and Post, F. (1980) 'Bipolar Affective Disorder in Old Age', *British Journal of Psychiatry, 136*, 26-32
10. Editorial (1979) 'Manic States in Affective Disorders of Childhood and Adolescence', *British Medical Journal, 1*, 214-15
11. Angst, J. (1978) 'Verlauf endogener Psychosen' in J. Finke and R. Tölle (eds.), *Aktuelle Neurologie und Psychiatrie*, Springer-Verlag, Berlin
12. Raskin, A., Boothe, H., Reatig, N. and Schulterbrandt, J.G. (1978) 'Initial Response to Drugs in Depressive Illness and Psychiatric and Community Adjustment a Year Later', *Psychological Medicine, 8*, 71-9
13. Paykel, E.S. (1978) 'Contribution of Life Events to Causation of Psychiatric Illness', *Psychological Medicine, 8*, 245-53
14. Hall, P. (1974) 'Differential Diagnosis and Treatment of Depression in the Elderly', *Gerontologia Clinica, 16*, 126-36
15. Mendlewicz, J. (1976) 'The Age Factor in Depressive Illness: Some Genetic

Considerations', *Journal of Gerontology, 31*, 300-3
16. Post, F. (1978) 'The Functional Psychoses' in Isaacs and Post, *Studies in Geriatric Psychiatry*
17. Cawley, R.H., Post, F., and Whitehead, A. (1973) 'Barbiturate Tolerance and Psychological Functioning in Elderly Depressed Patients', *Psychological Medicine, 1,* 39-52
18. Davies, G., Hamilton, S., Hendrickson, D.E., Levy, R., and Post, F. (1978) 'Psychological Test Performance and Sedation Thresholds of Elderly Dements, Depressives and Depressives with Incipient Brain Change', *Psychological Medicine, 8*, 103-9
19. Whitehead, A. (1974) 'Factors in the Learning Defect of Elderly Depressives', *British Journal of Social and Clinical Psychology, 13*, 201-8
20. Miller, E., and Lewis, P. (1977) 'Recognition Memory in Elderly Patients with Dementia and Depression: a Signal Detection Analysis', *Journal of Abnormal Psychology, 86*, 84-6
21. Nies, A., Robinson, D.S., Davies, J.M., and Ravaris, L.C. (1972) 'Changes in Monoamine Oxidase with Aging' in C. Eisdorfer and W.E. Fann (eds.), *Psychopharmacology & Aging*, Plenum Press, New York
22. Zung, W.K., and Green, R.L. (1972) 'Detection of Affective Disorders in the Aged' in Eisdorfer and Fann, *Psychopharmacology and Aging*
23. Cole, M., and Hickie, R.N. (1976) 'Frequency and Significance of Minor Organic Signs in Elderly Depressives', *Canadian Psychiatric Association Journal, 21*, 7-12
24. Post, F. (1975) 'Dementia, Depression and Pseudo-dementia' in D.F. Benson and D. Blumer (eds.), *Psychiatric Aspects of Neurologic Disease,* Grune and Stratton, New York
25. Hendrickson, E., Levy, R., and Post, F. (1979) 'Averaged Evoked Responses in Relation to Cognitive and Affective State of Elderly Psychiatric Patients', *British Journal of Psychiatry, 134,* 494-501
26. Jacoby, R.J. and Levy, R. (1980) 'Computed Tomography in the Elderly. 3. Affective Disorders', *British Journal of Psychiatry, 136*, 270-5

# 7 NEUROSIS IN OLD AGE

K. Bergmann

## Introduction

Does neurosis exist in old age? Why should we discuss it at all, how should it be defined, and if it can be defined, can we set up treatment aims that seem rational to us as therapists and also meet the needs of elderly people?

The existence of neurosis and emotional upset in older people can be challenged from several quarters. One such challenge is exemplified by the idea of the placid older person, the storms of life past, savouring the well earned tranquillity of a peaceful old age; in harbour, after the stormy ride of life, so to speak.

Less anecdotally, some support for the amelioration of neurotic disorders in later life is available from Karl Ernst,[1] who though not specifically studying the aged, did carry out a ten-year follow-up of neurotic out-patients, 37 per cent of whom were at least 50 years old before the follow-up was complete. Anxiety states were the most persistent and intractable, but other forms of disorder such as hysteria and depression improved or disappeared with the passage of time, and the general picture seemed to be that in old age the neurosis became milder.

Other studies which could contribute to this picture include that of Shepherd and Gruenberg,[2] showing steeply decreased claims on health insurance for neurosis and reduced out-patient attendance for neurosis with increasing age.

Kessel and Shepherd[3] showed a similar picture and even in general practice Shepherd *et al.*[4] showed that new cases of conspicuous psychiatric morbidity decreased with age as a proportion of all recorded cases. So is the problem of neurosis overcome by the mellow wisdom or reduced drive of old age? Optimists may choose to take the former view and pessimists the latter.

Surveys such as those reported by Kay *et al.*[5] do not suggest that either explanation is satisfactory; overall, about 12 per cent of people had moderate or severe disorder of a neurotic type. They also noted that a proportion of their survey subjects appeared to have developed neurotic disorder within the five years prior to their survey assessment.

The author's interest was stimulated by the apparent contradictions surrounding neurotic disorder in old age. The opportunity to study these problems further was afforded by carrying out an extension of the Newcastle survey employing the methodology developed by Kay and his co-workers.[5] Three hundred consecutive randomly selected respondents, between the ages of 65 and 80 years, without evidence of functional psychotic or dementing illnesses, were the subject of this inquiry.[6]

Using rather more inclusive criteria to define neurosis, 18 per cent of the sample appeared to have neurotic disorder of at least moderate severity and more than half of them appeared first to manifest their problems after the age of 60 years.

**Clinical Considerations**

The description of neurosis in old age that follows is based mainly on this study, though the author's views have been modified by later surveys carried out for different purposes and not yet published, and by the opportunity in recent years to treat patients with neurotic disorder in a district general hospital, in the setting of out-patient and day hospital care.

In order to provide a contrast with the onset of neurosis in later life, it is worth while examining the experience of long-standing chronic neurotics, as they come into their old age.

In old age the chronic neurotics, while still suffering from a multitude of symptoms mainly relating to an anxiety, did not suffer from any undue social or health stresses and, apart from an above-average degree of hypochondriasis, no greater maladjustment or discomfort than psychiatrically normal subjects.

These neurotics, often known to family doctors and clinics, were at peace with themselves with only hypochondriacal traits to keep their medical attendants and families on the alert! They could be said to be enjoying the best of neurotic ill health, having reached a balance which appeared quite satisfactory and best left undisturbed.

An example illustrating such a course of events was a 67-year-old widow: she had led a difficult life with marked psychosexual difficulties, money worries and fears related to childbearing. In her thirties she just experienced a moderately severe neurotic depression with severe feelings of tension and abdominal churning. As her children grew up, her menopause abolished the risk of pregnancy and the approaching Second World War brought prosperity back to her community; her symptoms became less severe. Though a pensioner and widowed, she enjoyed an extensive social life, going to the Townswomen's Guild, concerts, whist drives and clubs frequently. She still suffered from time to time moderately severe tension symptoms when some relatively minor events arose to disturb her obsessional habits and ordered existence. This lady was well adapted to later life and showed many of the characteristics that those who subscribed to high activity theories of adjustment in old age would associate with a satisfactory and normal life-style. The presence of neurotic symptoms, though still troublesome at times, in no way detracted from her enjoyment of life.

What is the situation of the late onset neurotic? Comparing their accounts of earlier life both with chronic neurotic subjects and normal subjects, an outline emerges. In childhood they resemble normal subjects more closely. They do not differ from them substantially in terms of reporting early neurotic traits, poor relationship with parents or differences in birth order.

However, in adult life differences from normal subjects emerge before the senium. Among the more important are reports of marital disharmony, psychiatric disorder in children, a tendency to marry at an early age, and to be of a lower social class.

Comparing them to the chronic neurotic group, they do not significantly differ in terms of the type of difficulties outlined above, though they do *not* over this period show any evidence of neurotic breakdown. In old age differences between chronic and late onset neurotics emerged. The latter differed from both chronic neurotics and normals, unfavourably in most respects; they were lonely, more isolated, had greater difficulty in sleeping, fewer hobbies and recreations. The stresses they experienced were more severe than either the normal or chronic neurotic groups encountered: including severe physical illness, heart disease, poor mobility and a low income.

It could be argued that these subjects were merely chronic neurotics with more stress, but it has to be emphasised that none of these subjects had in earlier life revealed any break of customary activity attributable to neurotic disability or symptoms: furthermore, their relatives and close friends, when they could be contacted, rarely saw them as being neurotic or nervous: their disability and symptoms being ascribed to ill health of 'old age' in the main.

An example of such a person can also be given: a lady of 76 experienced a series of falls with one or two blackouts, sciatic pains and unsteadiness of walk. When seen on the survey two to three years later her disability had become less marked. However, she remained very depressed, ruminating in an obsessional way about the losses of her life, especially the things she could no longer do. She also suffered from diffuse tension which was so bad that at times she felt she could scream. She had also contemplated suicide and felt that without her religion and friends she might well have made an attempt.

Her earlier life had been stable, hard-working, enjoying a happy marriage, bringing up two children, both alive and in touch with her. This lady was conscientious and very hard-working, and her inability to keep up with her own excessively high standards was emphasised by her attack of ill health. Her consequent reaction was out of all proportion to her disability, though she still maintained good relationships with children, friends and church, and was independent at home. She saw herself as worthless because she felt that she could not meet her own high internal standards.

In general, late onset neurotics could be divided into three groups. (1) The first group comprises those who gave an appearance of normality in earlier adult life, though some dependency and lack of resources was apparent, uncovered by a loss of support in later life. (2) In the second group are those people who, while showing good achievement in adult life, appeared to have been driven by strong neurotic forces such as obsessionality, guilt and anxiety focused on the need for approval. The loss of the ability to be 'superior' or earn approval and love by their achievements precipitates a neurotic reaction in later life. (3) The majority of late onset neurotics present a less clear-cut picture with some evidence of neurotic restriction in earier life, and some decompensation with loss of support and *raison d'être*, though it has to be emphasised that even this group were not seen as neurotic by their families or doctors.

## Personal Predisposition

It is evident that personal predisposition is perhaps the most important cause of breakdown in old age. Along with the others – stress, physical disease, cardiac disorder, loss of child, impaired self-care and isolation[4] – both necessary and sufficient causes of neurotic breakdown are provided in old age.

An examination of some of the factors associated with major abnormal personality traits identifiable in later life as being of some significance[7] is of importance.

Personality disorders of some severity are not easy to recognise, especially if they are unrelated to and independent of neurotic disorder.

In a random sample survey only 6 per cent of the population were found to be in this category. They could most readily be described as 'paranoid', 'explosive hostile' or 'inadequate'.

Neither of these groups of respondents suffered particularly in later life in terms of loss of interests and holidays and other features which might indicate maladjustment in old age: in many ways both life-styles, the surrender of the inadequate personality and the fight to the death often conducted by the paranoid personality seemed to produce satisfaction in facing life in old age when, as far as could be judged retrospectively, earlier adult life had not gone so well.

An illustration of the way an inadequate personality adapted well to the vicissitudes of ageing can be given: this example is of a single 71-year-old respondent who gave a 'senile' mumbling appearance without any evidence at all of the organic type of mental impairment. She had been all her life a shy unsociable woman, dependent on many relatives, never holding down a job outside the home, living, until death intervened, under the mother's domination, and after that with a succession of relatives on the same terms. Finally, she ended up with her younger sister and her brother-in-law, doing as she was told, expressing gratitude whenever it seemed appropriate, helping when required and apparently not arousing any resentment in the household and accepting her own situation equably and with good cheer. It could be said that people with inadequate personalities often accept with cheerful resignation the not infrequently unfavourable environment in which old people often find themselves; perhaps it might not be too fanciful to imagine that they have trained all their lives to face and accept a restricted final stage of their existence.

Diametrically opposed are the paranoid hostile personalities supported and energised by their hatred and anger, tolerating an isolation, even welcoming it, explaining away even their poor physical health as being due to machinations of their foes. Despair is not for them, for health, success and favourable conditions can be still hoped for, when their persecutors have been defeated!

An example of such a person was a lady of 66 years of age living in a cluttered-up room, eccentrically dressed in voluminously ill-fitting trousers revealing through their safety-pin fastenings large areas of pink knickers. She coped successfully with serious ill health, angina of effort, dyspnoea, ankle oedema and transient ischaemic attacks, letting rooms to two students and dominating an inadequate and simple-minded husband. Her attitude can best be gauged by quoting her: 'I don't like people, I'm aggressive, I prefer animals . . . ' She had quarrelled with all the local hospitals, family doctors and specialists, preferring at all times to dictate which treatment she should receive. This lady, had she heard one little voice, would have been labelled paraphrenic – nevertheless, she was tough and adaptive, dominating her environment without surrendering or retreating at all.

As with the inadequates, such older people seem to meet the insults and challenges of old age, but instead of losing hope or surrendering they go down fighting, but they take an extremely long time to do it!

The author's impression, purely on an anecdotal basis, is that the extremely old surviving independently in the community contain more than their fair share of tough independent rather prickly and paranoid personality types.

When we examine what personality traits are most associated with neurotic breakdown in old age then anxiety and insecure obsessional traits are of the most importance.

In early life these respondents already report more neurotic traits than others; mental disharmony is more evident in adult life, and long-standing gastrointestinal disorders are often associated with a long-standing history of tension feelings.

Nevertheless, there are those with this type of personality who do break down in old age, yet who have coped without obvious breakdown in earlier life. Such a diathesis may be at least to some extent genetically determined (Slater and Shields[7]), though it is not fully expressed until the neurotic reaction becomes evident in old age.

The insecure obsessional personalities, however, report poor parental relationships in earlier life, late marriage or staying single in adult life, psychiatric disorder in siblings and fewer social activities before retirement. Their history suggests that poor experiences in earlier life and associated restrictions throughout life might contribute to this set of vulnerable traits.

## Psychodynamic Aspects of Neurosis in Late Life

What sort of dynamic formulations are of use in understanding how such breakdowns in late life take place, given the types of personal vulnerability which are evident?

The vicissitudes of ageing are accompanied by many major threats – to life, to bodily function, to self-image and to social independence as well as to the life and health of significant others, spouses, children and friends.

Whatever stress is experienced in old age: be it bereavement, ill health, isolation or poor socio-economic conditions, elderly people can be found who do not develop severe anxiety, depression or other neurotic symptoms in the face of these events. Personal predisposition is therefore of importance in understanding the genesis of neurotic reactions in later life.

It is tempting to speculate that anxiety-prone traits, related to neurophysiological autonomic patterns of response, an early report of neurotic responses in childhood and the absence of any report of poor family interaction in earlier life, might indicate a genetic or constitutional tendency to react with more anxiety to external threats and life change. The fact that late onset neurosis is so highly associated with cardiac disorder may be related to a high level of underlying sympathetic over-activity.

On the other hand, the role of insecure obsessional traits associated with poor parental relationships and a tendency to marry later may indicate the influence of experience in earlier life. It is not easy to adopt classical dynamic concepts, such as the castration complex, into a working hypothesis, to explain how older people develop maladaptive reactions to threat. This has not prevented Schilder[8] from attempting to do this by postulating that, in old age, the castration complex transfers to the body as a whole!

The author has found Bowlby's[9] ethologically based model more useful. This model postulates that the young infant requires, at a critical period, stable maternal bonding in order to develop adaptive responses to life-threatening situations. Infancy and old age have this in common, in that they both represent stages when threats to life are commonest.

It is not unreasonable to suppose that some adaptive defect acquired early in life might not be manifested until the severe stresses of old age have to be faced.

Old age presents perhaps the toughest test of such learning. In old age itself 'learned helplessness' (Seligman[10]) and introjected anger may push neurotic reactions to the point of breakdown. The normal personality in old age is so remarkably individual that it is difficult to define systematically.

Though much has been made of the sufferings of the elderly, and at least 12 per cent suffer from moderate to severe symptoms of neurotic disorder and 5 per cent are clinical cases, they do not get treatment or help, and it is interesting to speculate why.

How does a person most often become defined as 'a case'? This is discussed by Goldberg[11] in some detail, citing Mechanic[12] and other authorities. Clinical experience and sociological findings do not suggest that the majority of psychiatric patients initially present asking for relief from their psychiatric disabilities. Those with neuroses usually present with failure of some aspect of their role at work or in the home with their spouse or children. Sanctions are threatened, the sick role is adopted, and after physical causes have been excluded (or missed), a psychiatric 'case' is defined.

How does the elderly person miss out on this chain? Why are older people suffering from acute neurotic reactions to stressful events not recognised as requiring treatment?

Perhaps the most important factor which makes the older person with neurotic disorder 'invisible' is that they no longer have, in most cases, a clearly defined role in society; the leader of the multi-generation family, the source of information, the teacher of craft skills – all these are roles in which, gradually, the old have become redundant.

From a medical view point the elderly have negative roles: not to be noticeably incontinent, not to wander abroad at night, not to have low standards of hygiene, not to create a risk with fire and gas. If such criteria applied in earlier life, neurosis would disappear from hospital and general practice records.

Associated with this question is the idea of 'normal' adjustment in old age. The correlates of successful ageing have been earnestly studied by sociologists. 'Activity' theorists have competed with protagonists of 'disengagement'. However, picking out in a simpler way how the normal person functions well in the day-to-day struggles of life and faces up to the stresses inherent in ageing has not been clearly outlined. What are the tasks by which we should assess success in the role of 'senior citizen'?

Their relationships with children and grandchildren must be one of the major areas in which older people retain a very clear role. With their own children the resolution of outstanding sources of anger and jealousy is an important job, and with grandchildren the ability to show feelings directly without worrying about issues of discipline and pressure of time can provide a new and age-related satisfaction. The pursuit of interests and good friendships for their own sake also call for well developed internal resources.

On the negative side the task of maintaining self-esteem and positive attitudes in the face of pain, disability and loss of function must be a major adaptive task.

Finally, facing death is an insoluble problem to which most people evolve only partially adequate strategies. Dependence, too, has a different meaning in old age. Physical ill health, poverty and lack of power may force many older people into dependent situations not of their own seeking, yet some very exacting and adaptive decisions have to be made by the older person. These might be formulated by the following questions: How much help do I need to accept to go on functioning in the best possible way? When I am receiving help from various sources, how do I co-ordinate it and remain generally in charge? How can I make those that help me feel that the experience is rewarding and pleasurable?

There are older people who deny, in the presence of severe disability, the need for any help. These can be called the pseudo-independent. They usually do receive help from an unacknowledged source, often a relative or neighbour, and will not accept help in any other form maintaining that they are managing well without any help, thank you! Such people often find a breakdown or crisis supervenes, leading to institutional care, due to the defective evaluation of their situation.

The greatest resource for community care of the elderly today is the family, yet the interactions of the older persons, their current stress and their families and friends have been strangely neglected. The situation is obviously a complex one, but at present there is room for simple observation and description of what happens between families and their older members with the passage of time, increasing dependence and ill health.

Several situations can be identified: for example the mother/daughter syndrome:[14] a daughter having lived all her life with mother, adoring, dependent, seeking mother's advice on all issues and obeying all commands issued by mother, faces a change in this stable benign tyranny due to illness, anxiety and depression coming on in the mother's old age. For the first time mother is put into the dependent and subordinate position, but the daughter is not ready to assume command. Tensions arise as the daughter assumes more and more responsibility in the absence of real power and resentments on both sides may be acted out in very childlike ways.

Other patterns include that of the 'fallen dictator' and 'power reversal'. The fallen dictator may be a powerful domineering husband and father, good at his job, well thought of at work, but tyrannical, overbearing and oppressive at home, having always maintained his command by instilling fear. When ill health and loss of income and work status remove the actual basis of power and when increasing demands for help at home undermine his position, his tyrannical attempts to retain command in the face of a changing situation may well create crises and rejection by the rest of the family.

The opposite case is that of 'power reversal', where, so to speak, the worm turns. The man in this case may have been described as an 'ideal' husband, constantly helping in the household, handing over the wage packet unopened, not smoking, drinking or going out with his work mates, constantly working to improve the house, taking pleasure in carrying out the wishes of wife and children. He is usually viewed, when not being ignored, with amused contempt by his wife and family. In old age, this invaluable family member may develop a life-threatening illness, heart attack or a cancer, and for the first time his every move and symptom commands the attention of the whole family. If he survives his illness he may have learnt one lesson: that he has the power to frighten, stir up and to be the centre of attention. This lesson once learned, he may be loath to return to his previous humble status. From that moment war is on, and the old person, by every childish and regressive means, attempts to retain power. I have even seen one such man threaten to kick his wife's most precious china cabinet to bits if she did not obey his wishes!

Behind such scenes many forces must be at work. Struggles for power, emotional and physical dependencies, methods of rewarding behaviour and roles whose basis lies in childhood fantasies and struggles, rather than in current reality.

There is a reluctance by many psychiatrists and physicians to see any place for psychotherapy with older patients. Any emotional crisis tends to be labelled as a 'social problem' and older people with depression, anxiety, hypochondriacal preoccupations and phobic states are offered home help, meals on wheels, voluntary visiting, outings and holidays. In fact, the only feature that most of these interventions have in common is that they don't require any medical input.

In many ways elderly patients with emotional problems fulfil the criteria for a good outcome: a good previous personality, a good work record and a stable family life and acute recognisable external stresses prior to breakdown. In addition, elderly patients are far too often 'managed' with toxic doses of psychotropic drugs when their psychiatric needs are identified, though the side-effects of psychotherapy can safely be presumed to be less noxious.

How then can psychotherapy based on a dynamic model be introduced into the care of the elderly? Should we model ourselves on the pattern of the psychiatric services in earlier adult life? This would entail departments of old age psychotherapy supplying individual and group treatments following special referral from general practitioners or other psychiatrists. Perhaps where great enthusiasm and the necessary resources exist such departments will arise.

The therapy for the elderly advocated by many American workers[14] is modelled on the standard office consultation in private practice. The issues dealt with are similar to those arising in earlier life, though the importance of loss, reminiscence of past events, physical illness and death are recognised.

However, in the context of the delivery of health care in the United Kingdom, primarily within the Health Service provisions, psychotherapy for the elderly has, in the opinion of the author, to be integrated with customary patterns of care. This presents several opportunities. Most elderly patients are assessed in a day hospital or in-patient unit by doctors, nurses, social workers, psychologists and occupational therapists. Potentially all these workers can become therapists, not because of their specialist training, but because of their human involvement with the older person.

During any assessment conference a dynamic formulation should be made involving, frequently, issues such as: bereavement, loss of status, loss of self-image, guilt and the problems surrounding dependency and impending death.

Families or close friends often have important and interdependent problems which have to be recognised. Failure to do so leads to a situation in which errors, mishaps and accidents often escalate; leading ultimately to an irreversible situation, beloved of the crisis intervention teams who now have something to respond to!

During the multi-disciplinary assessment, target areas for psychotherapy can be identified, for example abnormal mourning reactions requiring grief work, family rivalries in which childhood sibling rivalries may re-emerge, and intolerable fears and anxieties, both manifest and latent, which require a dependent relationship as a stage towards adjustment and coping. Often it is already apparent with which of the multi-disciplinary team the elderly person has engaged in offering their major emotional problems. The conference helps to define the targets of psychotherapy and the estimated frequency and duration of interviews.

Further review conferences allow the rest of the team to obtain feedback from the therapist and reciprocally to give support and, if necessary, effect modifications of therapeutic aims.

It is implicit to this type of psychotherapy that it is suitable to all diagnostic categories, neurotic, psychotic and organic. Diagnostic considerations mainly modify the complexity of the involvement and the degree to which families and friends may become the main focus of the psychotherapeutic involvement.

Group work also requires some modification for elderly patients. In general, rigidly transference-based psychoanalytically orientated groups do not seem to benefit elderly patients, who are less prepared to tolerate the high levels of anxiety which often occur in such groups. Quite often groups in old age can be made up of heterogeneous patients facing the same problem. Prolonged grief reactions, fears of facing the outside world and problems connected with loneliness and isolation are examples of commonly recurring themes.

Perhaps one important difference for the therapist in carrying out psychotherapy with patients in later life is the issue of dependency. Therapists working with the elderly have often to work hard to establish a relationship in which loving feelings and emotional needs can be expressed. The helpless elderly patients can once again feel they have power over someone and that their forbidden feelings of anger and self-destruction can be safely expressed.

In addition, the dependent bond between patient and therapist provides a place of safety from which the patient can dare to face external and internal threats.

Many elderly people who benefit from therapy are able to loosen their dependent bond and grow up again. Some tenuous link with a person or an institution may be necessary for a lifetime. Those fortunate enough to be visited by a member of the primary care team on a regular basis find this link meets their needs very well.

## Conclusion

Understanding neurotic reactions in later life, investigating dynamic issues and developing appropriate psychotherapeutic skills might be considered luxuries which the psychogeriatrician can ill afford the time to cultivate. But as fundamental cures for organic disorders are not yet available and even functional psychiatric disorder in old age pursues a remittent course, psychotherapeutic methods are often the main way to help elderly patients and their families. The alternative action to such help may be simply to arrange supportive measures, the provision of such supervisory visits, home helps, meals on wheels, day centres and clubs, and sometimes admission to residential care. While for some patients this form of help may be both appropriate and desirable, for others it may be useless or even harmful in that it renders the older person more dependent and helpless.

The major factor determining whether the elderly person gets appropriate help is the attitude of professional care-givers: the doctors, social workers, nurses or psychologists who may have contact with the elderly person.

If these professionals lack the ability to recognise emotional problems, formulate the dynamic issues and offer appropriate care, then their own anxiety may result in the offer of inappropriate, unnecessary or downright harmful support and services to the older person. This has economic implications, as we may well be spending a considerable sum on services that are mainly offered to allay the helpless feelings of care-givers.

The elderly person receiving help, given mainly to relieve the anxiety of the care-giving professional, is in many ways like the spoilt child, always dissatisfied and demanding more. The response in both cases could be epitomised by the remark 'And after all we've done for her . . . '

The most economical explanation of such situations is that the care-givers feel they have done more than enough, whilst the recipients feel that their most important, though often only implicit, needs are not being met. The majority of older people wish to remain independent, and understanding the emotional needs of other people and helping them to cope with their very stressful environment may need to be at the centre of many therapeutic programmes. The feeling that many sensitive and caring psychiatrists and other professionals have, when viewing old age psychiatry from without, is that it is a mechanistic pseudo-speciality in which people are moved around like counters and disposed of according to some sort of organisational scheme. The application of an understanding of dynamic issues to older patients and their families could not only benefit patients, but should help recruit the right sort of person to the field of old age psychiatry.

## References

1. Ernst, K. (1959) 'Die Prognoses der Neurosen', *Monograph Neurol. Psycbiat.*, *85*, Berlin
2. Shepherd, M., and Gruenberg, E.M. (1957) 'The Age for Neurosis', *Milbank Memorial Fund Quarterly*, *35*, 258-65

3. Kessel, W.I.N., and Shepherd, M. (1962) 'Neurosis in Hospital and General Practice', *Journal of Mental Science, 108*, 159-66
4. Shepherd, M., Cooper, B., Brown, A.C., and Kalton., G. (1969) *Psychiatric Illness in General Practice*, London
5. Kay, D.W.K., Beamish, P., and Roth, M. (1964) 'Old Age and Mental Disorders in Newcastle upon Tyne. Part I: A Study of Prevalence', *British Journal of Psychiatry, 110*, 146-58
6. Bergmann, K. (1971) 'The Neuroses of Old Age' in D.W.K. Kay and A. Walk (eds.), *Recent Developments in Psychogeriatrics*, British Journal of Psychiatry, Special Publication No. 6, pp. 39-50
7. Vispo, R.H. (1962) 'Premorbid Personality in the Functional Psychoses of the Senium. A Comparison of Ex-patients and Healthy Controls', *Journal of Mental Science, 108*, 790-800
8. Schilder, P. (1940) 'Psychiatric Aspects of Old Age and Ageing', *American Journal of Orthopsychiatry, 10*, 62-72
9. Bowlby, J. (1969) 'The Psychopathology of Anxiety: the Role of Affectional Bonds' in *Studies of Anxiety*, British Journal of Psychiatry Special Publication No. 3, pp. 80-6
10. Seligman, M.E.P. (1975) *Helplessness in Depression, Development and Death*, W.H. Freeman, San Francisco
11. Goldberg, D.P. (1972) *The Detection of Psychiatric Illness by Questionnaire,* Maudsley Monograph No. 21, Institute of Psychiatry, London
12. Mechanic, D. (1962) 'The Concept of Illness Behaviour', *Journal of Chronic Diseases, 15*, 189-94
13. Blau, D., and Berezin, M.A. (1975) 'Neuroses and Character Disorders' in J.G. Howells (ed.), *Modern Perspectives in the Psychiatry of Old Age,* Churchill-Livingstone, London
14. Post, F. (1950) 'Social Factors in Old Age Psychiatry', *Geriatrics, 13*, 576

# 8 PSYCHOTHERAPY FOR THE ELDERLY

Adrian Verwoerdt

Systematic research in psychotherapy is limited by the difficulties of applying theoretical concepts in ways that make it possible to measure them objectively. This is particularly true for psychotherapy for the elderly. A review of the literature shows that psychotherapy with the elderly is not conducted often enough in relation to the apparent need for it; that there is no basis for therapeutic nihilism; and that there is no systematised body of theoretical knowledge about the psychopathology of late life that would serve as a scientific basis for rational treatment planning.[5,8,18]

When designing a particular therapeutic approach, we must consider the following parameters: (I) The *topographical* factor, which refers to the structural aspects and answers the question, 'Where is something wrong?' (II) *The nature of the pathology*: what went wrong in that specific locus, and why? (III) The *therapeutic goal* is to intervene so that the structural or functional impairment in the topographical locus is alleviated. (IV) The *methodological* aspect refers to 'know-how': how to implement therapeutic objectives through specific techniques and interventions.

## I. Dynamic Psychopathology

### *A. Theoretical Constructs*

In the framework of dynamic psychopathology, we try to build theoretical constructs pertaining to the structure and function of the mind. Such theoretical constructs are useful only to the extent that they facilitate our understanding of behavioural-clinical phenomena.[17] Following a cybernetic schema, we discern *three basic functions* of the mental apparatus: (1) perception of incoming stimuli (input); (2) an adaptational function, which includes the autonomous and defensive ego functions (throughput); and (3) response patterns involving motor activity or behavioural patterns (output). (The autonomous ego functions include perception, thinking, memory, communication and certain neuromuscular capacities.) Certain stimuli, due to quantitative or qualitative factors, acquire the nature of stress; they cause tension which demands a solution, such as the removal of the stress. Motor activity aimed at removing the source of stress is a corrective (negative) feedback. On the psychodynamic level, we speak of adaptive coping. Maladaptive behaviour can be viewed as a case of positive feedback: the output has the effect of amplifying the input and increasing the stress. Defences can be adaptive (stress-reducing) or maladaptive (stress-amplifying). Intact ego function depends on intact brain functioning. Injury to the cerebral cortex means injury also to the ego functions.[2,3] When the cortex is impaired, both the ego's defensive (conflict-solving) capacity and the autonomous (conflict-free) functions (thought, memory, speech, perception, neuromuscular control, etc.) are affected.

Thus, in *dynamic psychopathology* we distinguish several interacting forces, including:

> the stress itself (for example loss of spouse) and the immediate emotional distress caused by it (for example grief);
> the defence mechanisms used to deal with the stress and its associated distress (for example denial); and
> the psychological and behavioural phenomena associated with such defences and coping behaviour (for example denial associated with grandiosity and hyperactivity).

In keeping with the above schema, *therapeutic intervention* can be grouped into three main categories, depending on whether the therapy is aimed at adjusting input disorders, at readjusting throughput disorders, or modifying the output. These three therapeutic categories, by and large, refer respectively to environmental support, psychotherapy proper and behaviour therapy.

### *B. Effects of Ageing on Coping*

The effects of ageing can be subsumed under two major headings. On the one hand, there may be a relative increase in the number and the severity of stressful experiences (various losses, physical illness, etc.); and on the other hand, age-related changes affect the ego's autonomous functions and defence mechanisms. The autonomous ego functions may be affected by neuronal impairments, by insufficient energy being available to them, or by withdrawal (decathexis) of the energy normally invested in the operation of these capacities. The latter is seen in various psychopathological conditions: decathexis of perception may lead to hysterical conversion symptoms, for example hysterical blindness; and decathexis of memory may cause amnesia.

With ageing, the usual ways of coping may have to be replaced by new techniques of adaptation. Aggressive mastery, for example, may be replaced by acceptance and the capacity to accommodate oneself to the inevitable without self-reproach or bitterness. High-energy defence patterns (the 'fight' response) include counter-phobic defences, over-compensation, obsessive-compulsive defences, the manic cluster (denial, hyperactivity and suppression through diversion), and the paranoid cluster (projection, hostile aggression against the externalised problem, or repeatedly fleeing away from the externalised threat). On the other hand, regressive defences (the 'flight' patterns, for example withdrawal) require less energy.[20]

### *C. Premorbid Personality Factors*

Patients whose premorbid personality is characterised by versatility in adaptation tend to have relatively less psychological decompensation following age-related losses. A premorbid behavioural style involving high-energy defences may be especially vulnerable to the psychotrauma of loss of mastery (for example from organic brain changes). Compulsive, rigid individuals are prone to react with profound anxiety when faced with the necessity of changing their habitual style and accommodating themselves to ego-alien constraints.[7,11] A possible link between certain premorbid personality traits (compulsiveness) and an increased vulnerability to depression is well recognised.

### *D. Interactional Effects*

The awareness of a loss produces the immediate response of anxiety or grief and mobilises specific defences, often precisely those whose continued operation is being threatened. An aggressive, ambitious person may try to defend against the threat of loss of control by becoming even more aggressive and controlling. The compulsive person may become more rigid and set in his usual ways. Inasmuch as the patient tries to meet the threat head-on, there will be more opportunities to experience failure, compounded by more anxiety, helplessness and feelings of shame and anger. A second vicious circle is set in motion when auxiliary defences, for example projection, are called into action. When this entails accusatory behaviour, the patient tends to alienate the very persons whose support is vital. If he tries to cope by withdrawal, the net effect will be similar: again the loss of external support. Still other vicious circles may be set in motion, linking up with those already there and adding to their momentum. The combination of persisting high-energy defences, intensifying negative emotions and weakening environmental support sets the stage for another systems breakdown, for example a new physical illness. In other patients, the course of events is less stormy, because they use defences that are less harmful, such as mild degrees of regression or denial.

## II. Treatment Goals

As mentioned above, treatment efforts can be categorised under three headings. (1) Therapy aimed at adjusting the input to the capacity of the mental apparatus comes under the heading of *environmental* support. (2) Improving the *functioning of the ego* itself comprises psychotherapy and psychopharmacology. This 'throughput therapy' includes two subgroups: treatment aimed at age-related autonomous ego impairments, and that aimed at the response to this stress (emotional distress and maladaptive coping). (3) Improving activity and action patterns comes under the rubric of *behaviour therapy* or behaviour modification. It is theoretically inaccurate and clinically unwise to select one treatment modality to the exclusion of others. Individual psychotherapy is a necessary element in the total spectrum of a comprehensive approach.

The conceptual framework of dynamic psychopathology forms a basis for a rational approach to treatment goals: *where* to intervene and the *direction* and degree of our intervention.

The overall objective is to re-establish in the patient a homeostatic equilibrium by implementing the following goals: (1) protective intervention: break up any vicious circle of interacting social, psychological and somatic factors; and adjust the environment to the patient rather than vice versa; (2) reduce the patient's need for capacities which are impaired; (3) restitution and replacement of impaired functions; (4) maintain residual functions; (5) treatment of distress to forestall further maladaptive defences; (6) replace maladaptive defences with those relatively less harmful.

## III. Psychotherapeutic Methods

### A. *General Principles*

1. Psychotherapy can be *defined* as the planned application, by a professional therapist, of specific psychological techniques to help the patient, by decreasing or removing psychological disability or misery, and facilitating optimal functioning. The basic skills involved include

the ability to make accurate observations of behaviour and to draw proper inferences from these; to synthesise the inferences in a tentative formulation which serves as a theoretical model and has implications for drawing up the treatment plan, and to observe the effects of implementing the treatment plan; and to use this feedback information for testing (confirming, refining, rejecting, etc.) the adequacy of the initial psychodynamic formulation. The goal of the therapist is, first of all, understanding. Whether or not he communicates his insights to the patient is a separate issue.[14]

2. *The Therapist-Patient Relationship: Obstacles.*

a. – *Patient Factors.*

(1) Because of sensory and intellectual impairments the patient has difficulty communicating and co-operating with the physician. It takes him longer to respond to questions, and he is more likely to forget treatment instructions. Therefore, one needs to talk more slowly (not necessarily louder), repeat questions and instructions, and write down advice.

(2) When entering into the doctor-patient relationship the patient takes with him characteristic attitudes and ways of relating to others derived from early past family experiences. Transference phenomena also vary, depending on the type of clinical setting and personality of the therapist. The latter may be seen as a parental figure, regardless of age differences. The concept of transference has practical implications, especially when negative feelings (hostility, guilt, envy) are being transferred. If one is alert to such transference distortions and tries to understand them, it becomes easier to tolerate and manage difficult behaviour.

(3) Other patient-related obstacles in therapy include physical and psychological *distress; socio-cultural factors* (cognitive impairments make it more difficult to bridge any socio-cultural gaps between patient and therapist); and *family pathology* (some families may deny the patient's illness, and cause the patient to go along with this attitude, or rebel against it by becoming unduly regressed – other families tend to infantilise the patient, thereby promoting premature regression).

b. – *Physician-related Obstacles.*

(1) The counterpart of the patient's transference is the counter-transference in the physician. It may represent a counter-role to the patient's transference. If the roles are fitting and appropriate, the

participants in the relationship have something to offer to each other. A counter-transference becomes a problem when it contains relatively strong neurotic components. Early emotional conflicts between the physicians and his own parents may be reactivated, causing specific counter-transference attitudes.

(2) Gerophobic attitudes on the part of the physician or his own unresolved fears of ageing and death make it difficult for him to treat elderly patients.[4] The obvious constraints in having to set limited therapeutic goals and the contemporary cultural emphasis on youth and attractiveness are added burdens.

c. —*Therapist-Patient Relationship: Optimal Attitude.*

(1) It is necessary to view disturbed behaviour as a malfunction of the total organism, just as one would regard physical symptomatology as a manifestation of malfunction of a particular organ. It is then easier to preserve an attitude of *detached concern* and to remain objective and helpful. This is especially useful when the patient is irritating or unresponsive to our therapeutic efforts. Whereas over-involvement is an 'occupational hazard' in the treatment of children and younger adults, the other extreme, defensive withdrawal, is more likely to occur in clinical work with old patients. An attitude of optimal empathy may be facilitated by keeping in mind that 'this old person once had the same age I have now'.

(2) A *realistic* approach to therapy is based on the recognition that no matter what symptoms the patient presents, there is always something the physician can do to give relief. One should recognise that attempts to alter long-standing character patterns are not only futile, but possibly harmful. The patient's behaviour should be met with an attitude of matter-of-fact acceptance; helpful assistance should never be accompanied by undue efforts to correct him, or by pointing out his deficiencies.

(3) A *consistent approach* combines gentleness and firmness, and makes it possible to set limits to undesirable behaviour (for example hyperactivity based on denial). Firm insistance, when used in the framework of a positive transference, may be effective, for example in certain withdrawn or underactive patients.

(4) Several types of therapist-patient relationships involve *dual roles* on the part of both participants. The patient may be older and may have had superior social or professional status; the therapist may feel constrained by some measure of awe, and the patient hesitates to settle in a dependent position. It is then useful to remember that a patient's

wish for support from a competent helper cuts across all ages and classes. Yet, some of this should remain tacit. On the surface level of the interaction, social amenities can be carried on in keeping with overt differences in status, class and seniority. The therapist may comfortably assume a deferential attitude, especially at the beginning and the end of the contact, and not challenge any pronouncements, but accept them with a mix of respect and matter-of-factness. And yet, somewhere during the interview he will shift his weight, easing both himself and the patient into the other dimension of their relationship, for example by giving specific advice or changing medication.

(5) *Getting and staying in touch.* Physical touch comes about in the most natural way, and reflects a basic way of getting in touch. Tuning in on the patient's emotional wavelength is another way of getting in touch. But, to stay in touch, one needs to keep the interview situation firmly in hand. There is only a limited place for non-directive interviewing technique and free associations. Goldstein uses the term 'communion' to indicate a state of solidarity between therapist and the brain-damaged patient.[9] Goldfarb[8] proposes that the patient be permitted to regard the therapist as a parent surrogate.

B. *Specific Techniques and Conditions*

The overall goal of re-establishing psychological equilibrium and maintaining contact with reality is achieved by implementing the following subsidiary goals.

1. – *Protective Intervention* requires therapeutic activism, somewhat in contrast to other psychotherapeutic approaches which emphasise a relatively non-directive posture and mental stance. The essential point is to be prepared to reach out for the patient and get in touch with him, rather than a passive wait-and-see attitude which would count on the patient to initiate contact. Many elderly patients are in trouble precisely because they have lost the ability to reach out to others, to stay in touch and maintain a relationship by efforts of their own.

In this framework of protective intervention, the therapist aims his efforts towards early recognition and correction of the many social and psychological decompensations, and the decline of physical health.

Furthermore, since the capacity for homeostasis declines, and the range of adaptation becomes narrower, one should not attempt to adjust the patient to the demands of the environment, but adapt the environment to the patient. When the environment (physical and social) has been adjusted to meet the needs of the patient, a state of equilibrium and health prevails. Concerning environmental support: abnormal sensory input may be quantitative or qualitative in nature. Quantitative input changes include sensory overload (for example chronic overcrowding) and sensory underload. Sensory deprivation or social isolation may be imposed on the individual (for example being alone in a hospital room) or may be the outcome of life-long character traits (for example schizoid isolation) or major psychopathology (for example depressive self-absorption). Qualitative changes in the input pertain to exposure to unfamiliar stimuli, such as sudden transfer to an institution.

2. – *Reduce the Patient's Need for Impaired Capacities.* The patient's ego may decompensate because of quantitative or qualitative changes pertaining to the individual's behaviour patterns, changes in the demands of performance and work, and modification in coping techniques (for example exhaustion from manic hyperactivity). On the 'output side' of our schema, we are concerned with modifying behaviour in such a way that it de-amplifies vicious circles (i.e. corrective feedback behaviour) and therefore becomes more personally satisfying and socially rewarding.[10]

3. – *Restitution and Replacement of Impaired Function.* Restitution of lost functions aims first at correction of medical and physical limitations. Since the problems of the bedridden or chair-ridden patient are far greater than those faced by the ambulatory patient, every effort should be made to preserve motility.[16] The increasing array of prosthetic devices is one of the exciting developments of modern medicine: glasses, hearing aids, dentures, artificial limbs, cardiac pacemakers, artificial hip joints, devices compensating for loss of sphincter control, etc. There are limits to the extent that prostheses can be used, particularly the constraints of the 'host' characteristics. Even an ideal prosthesis may no longer fit, because the infirmity of the prospective recipient does not support the prosthesis. From the utopian point of view, it is conceivable that almost all organs and body parts can be replaced by a prosthetic device, the exception being the brain. However, in the area of memory, thought and judgement, the patient may rely on others for support. These persons need to be well acquainted with the patient. This type of support, being an extra-corporeal cognitive prosthesis or memory device, cannot be expected from somebody who has known the patient only briefly.

4. – *Maintaining and Utilising Residual Functions.* For the patient to utilise his remaining functions fully, the physician must assume dual roles: being a personal physician to the individual patient and an organiser of health care functions by various professionals and agencies. Utilisation of residual functions is related to preventing regression and maintaining activity, and will be discussed below in further detail.

5. – *Treatment of Distress* is important for its own sake, and to prevent additional maladaptive defences.

a. – Generally speaking, to allay *anxiety* all the therapeutic principles underlying the optimal therapist-patient relationship must be observed. Appropriate dependency in the patient is therapeutically useful because it takes his attention away from anxiety-provoking concerns. Optimal regression, possible only in a firmly established therapist-patient relationship, is an effective antidote against anxiety and when the motive of anxiety is absent, maladaptive defences may be prevented from developing. When a positive transference exists, the patient looks forward to contacts with his therapist. Visits can be scheduled at regular intervals so that the patient has something definite to look forward to. In a hospital setting, rapport can be quickly established by frequent, brief visits (for example five minutes, three times a day, at the same time).

(1). *Depletion anxiety* refers to insecurity about the loss of external supplies and the possibility of isolation and loneliness. Its nature is not primarily in terms of a danger signal pertaining to unacceptable impulses from within, but corresponds with separation anxiety (depressive anxiety). The patient may not always be aware of the source of his anxiety, and therefore a careful exploration of his life situation is in order.

(2). Anxiety also may be generated by a shift from a perspective of self-confidence in the direction of *helplessness.* Anxiety pertaining to loss of control and mastery may be the result of decrements in the area of personal competence and autonomy. Since the associated anxiety is in terms of loss of self-confidence and shame, it is more difficult to obtain information than in depletion anxiety (where the patient can simply point his finger to an external problem). The patient is gently but firmly advised and assisted to get whatever medical examinations are in order: often elderly patients will resist having their alleged physical or mental defects examined. After the medical evaluation, it is also a frequent problem to get the patient to accept the recommended treatment. Here again, the positive transference in the relationship can serve its purpose.

Generally to reduce helplessness and enhance a sense of control, an 'obsessive-compulsive' behavioural style may be encouraged: preference for closure and predictability, avoidance of risks and uncertainty, and emphasis on schemas and schedules. Relatives can be advised that the patient's feelings of helplessness can be alleviated by anticipating some of his needs. This fosters a subjective sense of control and may prevent angry frustration, depression or shame. Patients handicapped by memory loss often have a relationship with one or more relatives in which the latter serve as an extracorporeal, prosthetic memory device. In contacts with such patients and their relatives, one can observe that whenever the patient's memory fails him, he sends out a verbal signal (a quick look) towards the relative, who then responds by filling in the necessary details.

(3). *Acute traumatic anxiety* may develop because of weakening of the ego's stimulus barrier. Normally, the ego is able to screen unwanted stimuli through selective inattention, external diversions, etc. In conditions of moderate to severe regression, the ego boundary becomes more penetrable, and the patient is more vulnerable to what may amount to a barrage of unwanted stimuli. This type of anxiety is characteristic of infancy, when the ego is immature, but may occur whenever the ego is relatively weak, as in old age. Milder cases show restless tension; more severe cases outbursts of rage, or defensive attempts to re-establish a stimulus barrier by withdrawal. Clinical management is supportive and includes drug therapy and environmental procedures. Supportive measures pertaining to environmental structuring essentially involve the providing of an 'ego prosthesis'. Such an artificial ego implies organising the patient's environment for him, with the spatio-temporal relationships of his milieu kept constant. The principle is that of sameness; by keeping the milieu constant, the sense of loss of mastery in the patient is minimised. Constancy can also be applied to arrangements of furniture, temperature, light, procedural methods, etc. Temporal constancy pertains to times of visits by the physicians, nurses, relatives, and so on.

b. – *Depression* usually has admixture of anxiety, and vice versa. Thus, treatment of depression will benefit anxiety, and again, vice versa. Depression is one of the causes of pseudodementia, but even if the dementia is organic, the admixture of depression will aggravate the symptomatology. It has been suggested that, since 25 per cent of all demented patients also have depression and, since depression may mimic dementia, all 'demented' patients should get a trial therapy with antidepressant medications.[16] More acceptably, whenever the diagnosis of dementia is uncertain, and there is evidence (such as the past history) to suggest the possibility of a depressive state, then a trial of antidepressant medications needs to be considered.

(1) *Depressive loneliness* is extremely common. Everywhere one goes in a chronic care facility, the question is heard: 'When can I go home?' This reflects the wish to be part of a familial, familiar setting – to belong – to be in touch with one's past and present self. Being uprooted in a strange place and cut loose from his moorings, the patient is as much alienated from his inner world as the world outside.

(2) Related to depression is *apathy*. Apathetic withdrawal may respond to an approach of appropriate stimulation. Many such patients are apathetic, because they prefer the gratifications of their inner fantasy world over those provided by the real world. The treatment approach includes elimination of possible iatrogenic apathy (for example excessive tranquillisation); remotivation, resocialisation and other group experiences; auxiliary therapies and appropriate stimulation involving antipsychotics or antidepressants. Apathetic *exhaustion* is treated by intensive support. The principle involved is to nurture and restore an organism whose inner resources and adaptive capacity are critically diminished (anaclitic therapy). This involves adequate treatment of any physiological disturbance and elimination of emotional insecurity by establishing a firm rapport and permitting the patient to become dependent on the parental figure of the therapist. Upon the return of emotional responsiveness one should not withdraw support, but maintain contact with the patient.

c. – *Shame and embarrassment* are the result of increased helplessness and decreased self-confidence. It especially occurs when dignity is lost. Dignity involves a special type of self-esteem: to be regarded well in the eyes of others. One loses dignity in public, not in privacy. To protect himself against possible ridicule and disgust from others, the patient may withdraw or defiantly use counter-phobic defences, but the price of intact dignity is loneliness, or the alienation of others.

The patient's need to maintain self-esteem requires a certain amount of denial on his part. This should be left intact, as long as it does not provide a serious risk to himself, others, or vital business matters. To protect dignity, it is necessary to provide the patient with the essentials of privacy, a space he can call his own, where he feels he belongs and can keep his belongings. Efforts aimed at reducing helplessness and promoting a sense of control will also enhance the patient's dignity. In protecting the patient's dignity, we protect his person, his self-image, his image to others and, in the final analysis, our own dignity.

d. – *Anger and aggressiveness*, being the result of frustration, occur under many conditions. Defensive hostility may be a cover for anxiety or depression; or, through an aggressive display, the patient may try to refute that he is helpless or shameful. In the wake of anger follows the conviction that the obstacle is out there – comforting thought, since attacking an outside threat is far simpler than coming to grips with the enemy within. The manifestations of hostility include vindictiveness; excessive complaining, but recalcitrance in co-operating with corrective intervention; lack of appreciation for what is done on their behalf; blaming others; gossiping, cursing and arguing; hitting others; spiteful acts (for example soiling themselves); etc. Management of these behaviour patterns requires an exploration of the role played by the premorbid personality and recent stresses, and a recognition that the hostile behaviour patterns are clinical manifestations of regression. The next step is, from a position of neutral objectivity and with an attitude of detached concern, to address oneself to the underlying concern and try to alleviate the stress. This may be a feeling of exasperating helplessness, shameful loss of dignity, bitterness about having been betrayed, or fighting against letting go for fear of being let down. In offering support, it is often necessary to use a special form of tact. The giving is not done openly, or formally, but tacitly and casually. This makes it possible for the patient to have his cake and eat it: he is receiving the needed supplies, and can still have his kicks by indulging in various protestations. By now, the stage for a collaborative relationship has been set, and one may attempt to deal with the disagreeable behaviour by setting limits. One method to convey to the patient the recognition that he is making some good progress, and that this testifies to his strength or courage. Again, the fact that the patient's strength has been 'borrowed' from the therapist is left unspoken.

6. – *Management of Maladaptive Defences.* Removing or mitigating maladaptive coping can be accomplished by alleviating the underlying anxiety that prompted the particular defence, or by replacing that defence with a more appropriate coping technique.[13] A patient's defences should not be exposed or removed without first ascertaining what he is defending against. A specific form of correcting maladaptive

behaviour is *behaviour modification.* The therapeutic goal is to modify maladaptive behaviour by extinction procedures, counter-conditioning, desensitisation, negative reinforcement and operant conditioning by token rewards. It seems that even in cases of moderate or severe organic mental disorders, behaviour can still be modified, provided the reinforcement is specifically suited to the individual patient.[1,12]

a. – *Defences Aimed at Mastery.*

(1) When the premorbid personality was characterised by *excessive self-reliance*, and when the patient now has developed actual dependency on others, for example for basic support in the areas of memory and conceptual thinking, this may set the stage for undesirable developments. The patient may react to increased dependency by becoming more controlling and defiant, and insisting that he can do without help from others. If the supporting persons try to correct him, he may react with anger, to the point where he might feel that others are against him. If, on the other hand, the supporting people happen to be absent or unresponsive, he will feel lost, confused and anxious.

2. *Paranoid behaviour.* When projection is the predominant mechanism, pathological suspiciousness and anger are the result. Clinical intervention is especially indicated when paranoid thoughts receive a charge of aggressive impulses. This mixture of paranoid suspiciousness and aggressive hostility is highly explosive.[19] There is a serious risk of violence aimed at disarming or destroying his alleged persecutors. The clinician must preserve an attitude of detached concern. Objectivity and neutrality are called for because of the patient's tendency to draw the therapist into the combat zone. Nothing is gained by trying to contradict the angry or paranoid patient or to correct his views. This will only confirm his belief that he is misunderstood by the physician. Nor is it therapeutically proper to agree with the patient. The correct response is to sidestep his attacks, to make clear that one will remain strictly neutral *vis-à-vis* the accusation, to acknowledge that the patient is having a hard time, and to indicate a willingness to help in accordance with the best of one's abilities.

b. – *Denial Mechanisms.* When dealing with denial, it is necessary to proceed with caution. One should never try to break through the denial by forcefully uncovering the underlying emotions. Blind adherence to the principle of confronting the patient with his mistakes or trying to 'correct' him is a caricature of therapy. Ventilation of concerns, however, is useful for specific emotions lying just below the surface, for example grief about loss, anger at medical personnel, or guilt about dependency. In patients with dementia the self is in a state of transition or crisis. Therefore, it is not always prudent to probe for thoughts and emotions, which do not contribute to the patient's sense of closure, such as current failures or past disillusionments. The tendency of many patients to make the best of it is not just a denial of some piece of reality. Rather, the attempt to seek out the sunny side of things in the here and now or, in retrospect, to beautify the past is nothing more than the work of that vital principle, hope.

c. – *Regressive Mechanisms*

(1) *Regression.* Optimal regression maintains a balance between the reduced assets (mental faculties) and the demand for performing tasks and activities. Therapeutic efforts include maintaining residual functions and preventing further regression through activity programmes. Daily activities can be structured according to a regimen that is consistent, predictable and sufficiently diversified. The activity spectrum should provide diversions and stimulation in keeping with the patient's personal wishes and remaining potential. Avoid the extremes of overstimulation and social or sensory deprivation, since each will exacerbate the symptomatology. Premature or excessive support has an adverse effect by promoting regression. Thus it is often difficult to stay on an intermediate course, avoiding on the one hand the extreme of insufficient support (which would create more anxiety), and on the other hand too much support (which would promote undue regression).

Motivation for activity must include a goal worth the effort. A patient may learn to walk again, but unless he has a motive for walking, he will soon abandon the attempt. The milieu of the average institution frequently offers little incentive to activity, thus fostering regression and deterioration. Self-care has appeal only to the extent that there is something to live for. The therapist and other treatment team members can become sources of incentive, by appropriately rewarding the patient's efforts. Activity is to be more than passive participation time-filling work. Therapeutic activity has purpose; the more completely it absorbs the patient's energies, the more beneficial it will be. When activities bring about contacts with other people, isolation is reduced.

In designing an activity programme find out the patient's interests; make a list of potential activities (indoors, outdoors) appropriate for the season; determine the patient's attention span for each of the activities; note the preferred time of the day and preferred sequence of activities; arrive at a mutually agreed regimen of daily activities; have the patient come back to report on the regimen. The need for an individualised approach to the patient is pointed up by the fact that for each individual, sick or healthy, the pattern of age-related decrements is specific and the rate of decline varies from one function to another.

(2) *Withdrawal* is maladaptive since it creates distance between the self and other humans and facilitates a final break with reality. If withdrawal is a life-long pattern (for example schizoid personalities), little can be done. In contrast to such characterological withdrawal, defensive withdrawal can be managed more successfully. First, sources of potential stress and distress should be eliminated to remove the risk of failure and shame. Second, approach of 'passive friendliness' should be tried in the context of brief, frequent visits. Third, one may try to change the withdrawn person into a hypochondriac; this would also apply to the schizoid cases. Bodily over-concern focuses attention on the real object of the body; the somatic symptoms provide a convenient alibi for mental failures; and the physical symptoms can set the stage for a traditional physician-patient relationship.

Although in most cases, hypochondriasis is the consequence of social isolation and self-absorption, in some instances the reverse is true. This happens when a withdrawn or autistic patient begins to turn his attention towards the real world. The first object encountered is his own body, which is like a bridge between the inner self and the outer world. The presence of physical complaints sets the stage for contact and interaction between the patient and another person. Hypochondriasis then represents a favourable development which may actually be encouraged.

*Hypochondriasis* refers to excessive preoccupation with the body or a portion of it, whether physical illness exists or not. The crucial element is bodily over-concern and self-absorption, at the expense of interests in other objects. The physical complaints do not have a symbolic or communicative function (as in hysterical conditions); nor do they reflect preoccupation with the physiological concomitants of an affective disorder (as in a depressive equivalent). Hypochondriasis may occur at any age, but is more common in late life. There are several reasons for this.

(a) *Chronic physical diseases* can serve as nuclei around which hypochondriacal concerns are precipitated. (b) It is fitting, in this context, to remind ourselves of the risk of *iatrogenic* hypochondriasis. The casual mentioning by a physician of a future complication may become a focal point around which hypochondriacal fantasies are elaborated. (c) *Object losses:* social isolation may set the stage for increased preoccupation with the one object that remains available: one's own body. Failure in the area of intimacy may, through distancing from people, bring about loneliness and isolation. (d) Failure in the area of generativity, through disengagement from work, may result in stagnation of the self. Thus the sick role becomes an alibi which removes responsibility for failure.

Because his self-absorption irritates and alienates others, the patient may experience further loss of affection, feel neglected and become disillusioned and bitter. The patient may stagnate in bitter resignation, or decide to do something about it. When such a psychodynamic constellation receives a charge of energy, the result may be aggressive vindictiveness (chronic complaints, fault findings; obstinate refusal to collaborate with others; vengeful sabotage of therapeutic programmes, etc.).

Successful management first requires a formulation of the specific psychodynamic factors playing a role. Any explicit interpretation of the dynamics, however, tends to be dismissed by the patient, and may in fact cause an exacerbation of the symptoms. Rather, it is wise to treat the symptoms without expecting that they will disappear. This is not therapeutic hypocrisy, but involves a dual communication, on two levels. On the superficial level, the patient and therapist are engaged in a traditional contract: to do something about the complaint. On a deeper level, however, there is a tacit understanding that, in order to maintain function and self-esteem, the patient needs his symptoms; that they are a form of coping, perhaps the only one available right now, and that the therapist is prepared to do the best he can to treat these symptoms, no matter how long it will take.

Some clinicians may decide to go along with the patient's contention that he is physically ill, giving him a particular diagnosis and a specific medication. Again, from a rational point of view, one would expect that such an accepting approach would give the patient what he wants. But sooner or later the patient returns, either with the old symptoms or with new complaints. The patient's first triumph was a pseudo-victory. The real winner was the physician, who had manoeuvred to set the stage for a traditional medical contract (the patient has an 'illness', gets medication and is supposed to get better) and had got the patient out of his office.

Therefore, when the patient asks for a diagnosis, it is prudent to circumvent this, and respond to the effect that 'Obviously you are having troubles. I am not certain about the real cause of the problem but I am glad to do whatever I can to help you.' Usually the hypochondriac will accept such a statement, which seems non-committal but at a deeper level is a statement of the physician's commitment.

Meanwhile, without some form of treatment, the patient may feel rejected because his symptoms are not taken seriously. Of course, many hypochondriacs do have actual physical disorders which would respond to appropriate medication. Drugs may be prescribed, provided one does not contribute to polypharmacy; and provided the drug has not already been used and contaminated by the patient's negative fantasies. It is better not to convey that the drug will be 100 per cent effective, but rather that it will help take the edge of the problem. This implies that the patient is to come back to tell how he is doing. This approach creates a 'no lose' situation: neither the doctor nor the patient will be forced into a position of defeat.

Next, the patient will test out the therapist's truthfulness. He may ask, 'How long will I need to take this medication: how long will I need to see you?' Giving an optimistic answer, to the effect that the patient may soon recover, is tantamount to failing the test. The patient knows full well that things won't happen this way. A pessimistic answer, to the effect that the condition is permanent, is also wrong, because the patient will wonder about the professional motives of having him come back for follow-up visits. The correct response is based on the recognition that the patient is not trying to find an objective piece of truth, but rather some evidence that the physician is 'true' to him. The patient may make the test of truthfulness even more difficult, for example by complaining that the time schedule for the follow-up visits is inconvenient. To avoid this trap, the therapist needs to face the situation with honesty, decide on the 'true-ness' of his commitment to the patient, and reiterate with firmness: 'It is important for you to come, and I expect to see you, even if it is inconvenient.' The tacit message here is: 'Look, in this relationship we aren't going to duck inconveniences, and you can expect the same on my part.' The point is implicitly made that the importance of the relationship transcends the magnitude of inconvenience. Thus one introduces a basic therapeutic ingredient: for the patient to carry on in spite of his problem.

When the patient improves, this should not become a basis for declaring him 'cured', or to have had 'maximum benefits' from the treatment – and then terminating the treatment programme. Rather the improvement indicates that the treatment regime is sound and must be continued. By the same token, one would not stop giving insulin to a diabetic because he is responding well. As the patient returns, more emphasis may be directed toward problems related to people, external interests or outward-oriented activities.[12]

*Some Comments on Organic Mental Disorders*

Our definition of 'psychotherapy' (see above) points up the unique difficulties of applying this to patients with dementia. The 'application of psychological techniques' is based on the premiss that there is a suitable medium for transmitting therapeutic information. In dementia, however, this very medium (the communicative channels) is impaired. Secondly, the target towards which psychological techniques are directed to 'decrease or remove psychological disability' (the brain) is afflicted with permanent damage. To deal with these difficulties, it is necessary to view psychotherapy as *therapeutic communication.* And, when we speak of individual psychotherapy with senile dementia, it is more useful to think of this as: how to be psychotherapeutic with the individual dementia patient.

In psychotherapy with dementia patients, *transference* is not interpreted as in insight-oriented therapy. Transference usually goes along with an observing ego capable of discerning the 'as if' element in comparing a person in the present with one in the past. The dementia patient loses the ability to compare; there is an impairment of the observing ego: the ego can no longer detach itself from an experience, but becomes an active participant. Transference phenomena in these patients may develop instantaneously.

A 78-year-old woman's first statement to me was: 'Your wife has died.' There were several levels of meaning to this; at that moment of getting acquainted, the relevant idea was that if my wife was dead, we would be 'available' for each other – and that for this to be on her mind, she probably liked me: somebody to be with. She provided further evidence of this, saying: 'And she over here [the nurse] is your daughter.' Through this concrete transference, she expressed a specific feeling: that it was like a family here – that she felt at home.

Other transference distortions refer to the environment. When patients say that this place here is a hotel, school, courthouse or jail, this is not just 'disorientation for place and person'; rather, such a misidentification is often a concretised representation of an inner feeling state.

Later, the above patient stated, 'Now you and I are married' – ideas of permanence and closeness are expressed through the concept of marriage. Proceeding along her line of thought, I asked if she was going to be in the family way – 'Oh, yes – we'll have children but not now – in a few years' – in other words, the closeness between us will not end for quite a while.

*Language and communication:* frequently, taking the patient's statements at face value is not conducive to understanding. Yet, for these patients, the very existence of any 'true' communication would be, in and of itself, therapeutic: it keeps the patient in touch with reality. The question is: how do we make sense out of the patient's frequently chaotic thoughts, and how can we enter into his world and speak his language? The chaotic thinking in dementia is the result of an impaired abstract capacity (in psychodynamic terms, regression from secondary to primary process thinking). The thought processes are similar to those observed in dreams. The fact that all of us 'share' this primary process thinking may be a basis for understanding the patient's thinking. For the actual clinical situation, some practical guidelines are suggested by the very nature of primary process and the consequences of impaired abstract capacity.

In *paleologic thought*, a common predicate leads to the establishment of an identity of two nouns (subjects).[6] The above 78-year-old patient called her ward physician 'a preacher'. When asked what preachers do: 'They preach about heaven – that is nice.' That was also the way she saw her physician. Cognitively, she was unable to recognise him as a member of the general category of 'physicians', but emotionally, she received from him 'good feelings' and associated these with the preacher she had known so long. Technically, then, the first step is to observe the concrete idea presented (preacher). Next, we obtain the relevant attributes of this subject (preacher = man in authority + nice). Third, we see if this key fits other locks: 'Man in authority who is nice' also fits the patient's doctor.

The primary process does *not know of a negative, a possibility or conditionals.* The most frequently asked question by patients on a geropsychiatric in-patient unit is: 'When can I go home?' Trying to give a logical answer (in keeping with secondary process and reality orientation) often appears to leave the patient distressed. Further enquiry may reveal that he does not even know where his home is; or he talks about a home where he lived long ago. The point is that the question is a statement; the word 'when' means 'now'; and 'home' stands for 'at home'. Thus, the translation produces: 'I do not feel at home here' – or 'I don't belong here – I don't belong – and I feel lost.'

In the primary process, there is no *time sense.* In an interview, a patient may move back and forth through the time tunnel without constraints. To tell him: 'Today is [day, month, year] and we are at [institution, city, state], etc.' might not be meaningful because he does not have the temporal structure into which to fit this information.

Since impaired abstract capacity leads to inability to *account to oneself for one's acts*, it is not fruitful to ask the patient why he did this or that. One patient, when asked why she kept having trouble with her wheelchair, responded: 'I have not had lunch yet.' This also illustrates projection and condensation: embedded in her response is the accusation: 'You don't feed me – that's why I can't do things around here.'

Dementia patients have *difficulty getting started* on a task, taking initiatives or making decisions. Once they are put on the right track, though, they may keep going, sometimes to the point of perseveration. Open-ended questions confuse the patient. It is useful to make contact by focusing on a concrete item, for example dress or physical symptoms. Of all the objects in the patient's world, his body remains the closest one to him.

*Inability to keep in mind various aspects of a situation simultaneously:* the patient can see the individual tree, but cannot conceptualise the forest as an idea. If the nurse gives him a shot, 'She hurts me – hurting me is what my enemy does – so she is my enemy.'

Another pheneomenon, relevant to this context, is that the patient will end up rambling. When he sets out, in a statement, to make a point, he can't allow himself to digress (for example by adding descriptive details), because during the moment of digressing, he loses sight of where he was heading. He never gets to the point, never makes his point. To prevent such derailments, the therapist should firmly but gently intervene in the rambling and keep the patient on the right track. It is crucial to do this in a good-natured, non-critical manner lest the patient should feel put on the spot and is forced to face his failure.

The patient falls back on the so-called *emotional attitude.*[9] He responds to stimuli on the basis of the pleasure principle: either pleasant (good) or unpleasant (bad). Example of dialogue: Who is that person (a nurse)? 'She is nice.' What kind of things does she do? 'She is nice to me.' How? 'She gives me baths and foods.' Such a patient can enumerate certain qualities of the nurse but cannot recognise her as a member of a conceptual category ('nurses'). Since the ability to express emotions remains relatively intact, it is a good technique to tune in on the patient's emotional channels, rather than something abstract.

During interviews, avoid 'conceptual' questions which would put the patient on the spot and cause a catastrophic reaction. A 79-year-old man showed clinical evidence of some loss of the capacity for conceptual thinking. When asked about the year of his son's death, he knew that this was twenty years ago. But after repeated questions about what year it actually had been, and after establishing what the present year was, he was not able to subtract twenty years from that. Instead, he added them on to the present year, which brought him close to the end of the twentieth century. At this point, he revealed perplexion and profound anxiety. He then mumbled: 'Or 2000?' The patient gives a wrong answer, is aware of his inability to perform accurately, develops profound anxiety, and becomes totally unable to perform.[15]

Decrease fear of the unknown by focusing on body sensations and physical symptoms. Many patients start off an interview by presenting physical symptoms seemingly bizarre or inappropriate. These should not be dismissed as irrelevant because it may be the patient's only way he can still make contact.

## Summary

In summary, the psychotherapeutic treatment of the elderly utilises regular methods as in younger adults, but, because of the probability of impaired autonomous and defensive ego functions, along with frequent physical impairments and social-environmental changes, it needs to be tailored to fit the individual. If this is done, help can be rendered effectively. Specific therapeutic goals and methods involve protective intervention, reduction of the patient's need for impaired capacities, restitution and replacement of impaired functions, maintenance of residual functions, treatment of emotional distress and replacement of maladaptive defences with less harmful ones. In addition, in the case of dementia, an understanding of primary process thinking may be useful.

## References

1. Ankus, M., and Quarrington, B. (1972) 'Operant Behavior in the Memory-disordered', *J. Gerontol, 27*, 500-10
2. Von Bertalanffy, L. (19766) 'General System Theory and Psychiatry' in S. S. Arieti (ed.), *American Handbook of Psychiatry*, Basic Books, New York, vol. 3, Ch. 43, pp. 705-21
3. Brosin, H.W. (1952) 'Contributions of Psychoanalysis to the Study of Organic Cerebral Disorders' in F. Alexander and H. Ross (eds.), *Dynamic Psychiatry*, University of Chicago Press, Chicago
4. Bunzel, J.H. (1973) 'Recognition, Relevance and De-activation of Gerontophobia', *J. Am. Geriatr. Soc, 21*, 77-80
5. Butler, Robert N. (1975) 'Psychotherapy in Old Age' in Arieti (ed.), *American Handbook of Psychiatry*, 2nd edn, vol. 5, Ch. 42, pp. 807-28
6. Von Domarus, E. (1944) 'The Specific Laws of Logic in Schizophrenia' in J.S. Kasamin (ed.), *Language and Thought in Schizophrenia*, University of

California Press, Berkeley, pp. 104-13

7. Gianturco, D.T., Breslin, M.S. Heyman, A., Gentry, W.D., Jenkins, C.D., and Kaplan, B. (1974) 'Personality Patterns and Life Stress in Ischemic Cerebrovascular Disease. 1. Psychiatric Findings', *Stroke, 5,* 454-60
8. Goldfarb, A.I. (1967) 'Geriatric Psychiatry' in A.M. Freedman and H.I. Kaplan (eds.), *Comprehensive Textbook of Psychiatry*, Williams and Wilkins, Baltimore, Ch. 47, pp. 1464-87
9. Goldstein, K. (1959) 'Functional Disturbances in Brain Damage' in Arieti, *American Handbook of Psychiatry*, vol. 1, Ch. 39, pp. 770-93
10. Katz, L., Neal, M.W., and Simon, A. (1960) 'Observations of Psychic Mechanisms in Organic Psychoses of the Aged' in P.H. Hoch and J. Zubin (eds.), *Psychopathology of Aging*, American Psychopathological Association Proceedings
11. Kiev, A., Chapman, L.F., Guthrie, T.C., and Wolff, G. (1962) 'The Highest Integrative Functions and Diffuse Cerebral Atrophy', *Neurology, 12*, 363-85
12. Mueller, D.J., and Atlas, L. (1972) 'Resocialization of Regressed Elderly Residents: a Behavior Management Approach', *J. Gerontol., 27*, 300-92
13. Verwoerdt, A. (1972) 'Psychopathological Responses to the Stress of Physical Illness', *Adv. Psychosom. Med., 8,* 92-114
14. Verwoerdt, A. (1976) 'Psychotherapy and Sociotherapy' in *Clinical Geropsychiatry*, Williams and Wilkins Baltimore, Ch. 11, pp. 132-46
15. Verwoerdt, A. (1976) 'Schizophrenic and Senile Psychoses, in *Clinical Geropsychiatry,* Ch. 15, pp. 185-99
16. Wells, Charles E. (1977) 'Diagnostic Evaluation and Treatment in Dementia' in C.E. Wells (ed.), *Contemporary Neurology*, F.A. Davis, Philadelphia, vol. 15, Ch. 12, pp. 247-76
17. Wang, H.S., and Busse, E.W. (1971) 'Dementia in Old Age' in Wells, *Contemporary Neurology*, Ch. 9
18. Weinberg, Jack (1975) 'Geriatric Psychiatry' in Alfred M. Freedman, Harold I. Kaplan and Benjamin J. Sadock (eds.), *Comprehensive Textbook of Psychiatry*, 2nd edn, Williams and Wilkins, Baltimore, Ch. 49, pp. 2405-20
19. Wolk, R.L., Rustin, S.L., and Scotti, J. (1963) 'The Geriatric Delinquent', *J. Am. Geriat. Soc., 11*, 653-9
20. Zetzel, E.R. (1965) 'Dynamics of the Metapsychology of the Aging Process' in M.A. Berezin and S.H. Cath (eds.), *Geriatric Psychiatry*, International University Press, New York, pp. 109-19

# PART THREE: SERVICES

# 9 WHAT IS A 'SOCIAL PROBLEM' IN GERIATRICS?

R.V. Boyd

The concept of health embodies not only the absence of disease, but the presence of a positive sense of well-being. A healthy person functions well in both bodily activity and social relationships; conversely, an unhealthy person is likely to have altered personal relationships. The effects on social functioning may be slight, temporary and easily compensated, or they may be major, permanent and irretrievable. Every ill person has a social problem and the severity needs assessment and appropriate interest and action.

Social problems associated with disease are likely to be more profound the longer the illness lasts and the greater the disability. The elderly have a high incidence of both chronic illness and disability and consequently the geriatrician as part of his daily practice is concerned with many patients who have social problems associated with their illness.

## Type of Social Problems

At any age such problems as homelessness, poor housing and unemployment are the province of the social worker; while the elderly may be affected seriously by this type of circumstances, the implications for health, although important, are indirect.

The social problems considered in this chapter are those which stem from physical illness of the elderly individual, together with those aspects of mental ill health which are the legitimate interest of the general physician.

## What is 'Health' in an Old Person?

For a younger adult health is obvious, but so many negative attitudes abound that some comment is necessary.

The gradual deterioration of function with increasing age is so widely perceived and so expected that all deterioration in function in an elderly person tends to be attributed to age. There is a logical solecism here of the type:

> Dogs have four legs; cats have four legs; therefore cats are dogs. Senescence produces deterioration in function, *ergo*, deterioration in function in the elderly must be due to old age.

Yet disease produces deterioration in function and is easily confused with senescence. The importance of this distinction is that much can be done to alleviate or even cure disease, while nothing can be done to reverse senescence.

In practice there is only one safe approach to the elderly, and that is to expect a fit old person to be personally independent, continent and rational; only in the extremes of age are significant physical or mental limitations found which might be attributed to ageing. Even then numerous exceptional individuals surprise by their memory, wit and nimbleness, and it is unsafe to attribute major disability to senescence at any age. The extremes of age are still largely uncharted territory in relation to the limits of physiological change, and it is unwise to dismiss limited function as due to incurable senescence. Indeed, increasing age predisposes increasingly to pathological processes, hence the need for more than usual care in the very old.

Unfortunately most people, both professional and lay, take a passive approach to disorders in the elderly. People tend to expect the doctor, when called to see an ill or disabled old person, to attribute the problem to 'old age', and any other opinion may even be resented. In the South-West of England there is an expression 'The age is there,' and when an old person has a health problem a doctor can shake his head wisely while solemnly pronouncing these words, and obtain approving acceptance by interested parties, including the patient, regardless of the pathology present.

Under these circumstances, suggestions of investigation and treatment are resisted; the geriatrician needs to overcome these negative attitudes before beginning to help the elderly patient, and it is often a long process for the geriatrician to establish his own credibility and engender a positive approach. Yet when this happens it will become routine for an old person with problems of mobility, mental change or incontinence to be assessed for disease and for appropriate remedial action to be taken.

**Atypical Disease Presentation in the Elderly**

Disease in younger adults usually produces characteristic symptoms and signs by which a particular disease is recognised; if a diagnosis is not achieved on initial contact with the patient, the symptoms and signs are used as a base for further investigations and action. The patient who is ill without symptoms and signs directing a course of action towards a specific diagnosis is unusual.

Medical training is orientated towards recognising these patterns, and physicians have developed ways of tackling, say, chest or abdominal pain in order to establish or confirm the diagnosis.

Functional disability due to disease attracts little medical interest, which is concentrated upon the specific features of the disease; thus the referral letter about a younger patient with suspected myocardial infarction is likely to discuss the features of the chest pain, but is unlikely to mention whether the patient can walk to the toilet or feed himself.

The elderly may experience the same symptoms as younger people, but often the specific features of disease are missing; there may be gross underlying pathology while the typical aspects do not develop – for example, myocardial infarction is often silent[1] and peritonitis may be painless.[2]

In the absence of particular symptoms, the elderly often display only the non-specific features of disease, i.e. they fall or take to their bed, become incontinent or exhibit mental disturbances. This triad of physical disability, mental disability and incontinence is the common pathway of disease in the elderly; all disease can present in this way and, conversely, the elderly person manifesting these features can have virtually any pathology. To the doctor who has been educated only in the classical disease-picture of the younger patient, the elderly person presenting without these disease-pictures can have a disorientating effect; the doctor may draw the apparently logical conclusion that because the specific symptoms are absent, the patient cannot have a particular disease.

This failure of the elderly patient to fulfil the doctor's expectation of disease is of considerable importance. Hospital services are geared to tackling disease with particular symptoms, and the presence of these symptoms is the means of gaining access to hospital facilities. A symptom such as chest pain acts as a password to gain access to hospital facilities. The absence of such a symptom in an ill old person means that he has no such 'Open Sesame' to health services.

The position is further complicated by the tendency of old people to have several, or many, disease processes at once. To dissect the multiple strands of diseases and their relative effects upon an individual patient requires patience and application founded upon interest; this basic interest is often lacking in the doctor because the patient does not fit into the traditional pictures of disease which the doctor has learnt.[3]

The passive approach to disability in the elderly can be emphasised by comparison with attitudes to the minority of younger patients who present with non-specific features. When a younger adult develops a significant limitation of activity it will be investigated and treated even though there are no focal features to attract attention; if recovery is complete, all well and good, but if there is residual disability positive plans will be made to cope with that disability. In an old person, equivalent disability may be dismissed as 'old age' and the opportunity for diagnosis, treatment and detailed future planning may be lost. Support systems for a limited old person are instituted without exploring diagnosis and treatment.

So what about the old person, presenting with his triad of non-specific features? The existence of the patient cannot be denied, nor that there are problems over the care of such an individual, but he is denied access to health facilities. The common way to dismiss the situation medically is to apply the label 'social problem'. It is an obvious fact that there are social difficulties over the care of the old person who has developed mobility problems, mental symptoms or incontinence, and under the rubric 'social problem' those problems are made the responsibility of someone else – the social worker. The underlying medical needs for diagnosis and treatment are ignored.

This sequence of events is unlikely in an acute illness, when a fit and active old person changes dramatically to become bedfast, delirious or incontinent; the medical content of such change is usually easily seen. In the illness of gradual onset with gradual progression over many months, however, the medical element is disguised. The patient/client may present with gradually decreasing capabilities to the Social Services Department and compensatory increments of domiciliary services are instituted under the guidance of the social worker. When the stage is reached that the domiciliary serves are insufficient to meet the needs of the patient/client, the social worker has little alternative but to seek admission to a residential home. Theoretically, at every stage in this sequence medical care is available, but if the perception of need is in the terms of a 'social problem', useful medical input does not occur.

**Effects on Social Services Departments**

The inference from the argument so far is that Social Services departments carry an inappropriate burden in providing services for the elderly disabled who have potentially treatable medical problems. The presence of many unrecognised medical problems amongst the elderly is well documented[4] and the logical conclusion is that the need for domiciliary services and residential care would decrease if these medical conditions were treated appropriately. The validity of this conclusion has yet to be tested.

In clients presenting for admission to residential accommodation, many medical problems are found.[5] Figures on death rates after admission to residential accommodation are difficult to obtain, but studies from Coventry and Edinburgh show an excessive mortality.[6,7]

These results support the contention that medical problems in the elderly present in the guise of social problems, and that social workers and the staff of residential homes are left to cope with what, in reality, are medical problems; with the best will in the world, these personnel and facilities are not equipped to provide health services.

**Sickness Roles and the Elderly**

The sick younger person manifests certain features of disease and its consequences which are tolerated and approved. For example, a sick person of working age is allowed to take time away from work and to receive sickness benefit and other supports, while retaining social approval. If a person is abusing this system there is social disapproval and legal sanctions may be applied. For all young patients there is loss of status, restriction of activities and at least some loss of income.[8]

The situation is obscured in the elderly who are retired and who are generally expected to need support simply by being old. When disability occurs in the elderly there is usually no loss of income within a family (indeed in the United Kingdom the Attendance Allowance paid to relatives who care for the elderly may increase income) and other consequences of illness are less obvious. Families tend to expect an old person to be dependent, and rally to give social and nursing support. For the elderly, therefore, the context of the sick role is different from younger adults and there is less pressure to overcome sickness and disability; relatives are under a greater sense of duty to provide help.

**Do Relatives Fail in their Responsibilities to the Elderly?**

It is widely believed that relatives fail to meet their responsibilities to old people. 'Children' of octogenarians and nonagenarians are themselves often sixty or even seventy and are limited in the support they can give. Present-day families in Western society tend to be small, with only a few relatives in any one family; in addition, the mobility of present-day society means that a family is not localised to one town or village but scattered widely, perhaps over the globe. Even a few minutes' travelling distance makes support difficult; this is especially true when there are other family or work commitments.

Two studies have attempted to answer the question whether families face up to the responsibilities of looking after older relatives. In Edinburgh[9] a series of 1,500 admissions to a geriatric unit, retrospective and prospective, was published. There were 1,115 discharges which were assessed in the light of what was considered to be a reasonable burden that relatives could be expected to cope with in the light of other responsibilities, such as the presence of young children and the need to pursue outside employment. Of these 1,115 discharges, in only 12 were the relatives felt to be unreasonable in not providing support, barely more than 1 per cent. In contrast, there were many families who assumed major burdens in relation to their other commitments; five times as many relatives undertook 'unreasonable' home care of the elderly who had major disabilities as refused to take what was considered to be reasonable responsibility.

A Glasgow study confirmed these findings when Isaacs assessed 280 referrals for admission.[10] While 7 patients actually refused help from relatives, only 11 relatives were judged to be giving inadequate support. When these were interviewed, it transpired in every case there were major factors from the past which had hindered relationships, for example alcoholism, prostitution or marital disturbances. In only one case amongst the 280 was it felt that the relatives failed in their responsibilities and wished to enjoy their own social life in preference to supporting an old person in need.

Surveys of the elderly in the community[4] have shown a high incidence of medical and social need which is not only unmet by statutory services but which had been unrecognised. The main strain falls upon relatives. In departments of geriatric medicine that operate 'holiday' relief services, some insight is obtained into the degree of support that individual families give to the disabled elderly. In these schemes, the elderly disabled person who is normally cared for at home is admitted to hospital while relatives have a holiday (similar schemes for the less disabled are operated by local authority Social Services departments). Those old people admitted to hospital under this arrangement are often among the most disabled in the ward and yet are nursed at home for most of the year.

## Problems over Discharge from Hospital

Problems over discharge from hospital are often regarded as 'social problems'. This term is used to cover situations where the old person is fit and active but homeless, poor or lonely, and also situations in which the old person has residual medical problems.

When discharge difficulties are encountered, one solution often considered is placement in permanent institutional care; this may be in a residential home, a long-stay hospital bed or in a private residential home, depending upon the subject's capabilities and financial resources. The temptation to provide institutional care is considerable because not only is this so often what the patient and the relatives expect, but also because it relieves those associated with the elderly, including the doctor, of the need to cope with the anxieties and difficulties inherent in supporting the old person at home.

Admission to an institution where a vacancy is available is the line of least resistance, since support at home needs effort and worry, often over a long period, for relatives and friends and professional advisers. Fine and dispassionate judgement is needed in such decisions before advising the patient/client and the relatives; often the correct course of placement and support at home is in conflict with merely superficial assessment of the course of action to place a client in residential care. This is particularly so when a patient is about to leave hospital and placement in a residential home seems a simple and secure decision. Many old people with permanent and incurable disabilities will be at risk if sent home, yet the alternative of placement in institutional care takes away what independence they have and risks the consequences of institutionalisation.

In consideration of discharge, there are several commonly recurring reasons given for avoiding the decision to return home. There are, for instance, the risks of falls or of loneliness, or the fact that the person's home is too large. Commonly a large house is said to be too taxing for a disabled old person to cope with; yet it is perfectly possible for a disabled person to live in one room, whether that one room comprises the whole of a one-room flatlet or is one room in a large mansion. It is feasible to live in a single room used as a bed-sitter whatever the size of the overall accommodation, if necessary, with a commode, given appropriate support with shopping, housework, cooking and emptying the commode; even in the absence of relatives, in the United Kingdom the domiciliary services should be sufficient to meet such needs. Sometimes the modified arrangements that may later be necessary in terms of sale of the house with removal of the old person to a more suitable flat can be negotiated after discharge to a one-room life; such major modifications can be implemented after return home. The local authority Housing Department usually takes a helpful attitude and will exchange the house of a patient (which will provide accommodation for a larger family) for a flatlet.

Loneliness is a problem experienced by many old (and younger) patients in their own homes. Considering discharge from hospital, it is not reasonable in the light of a shortage of in-patient facilities to defer discharge simply on the grounds that an old person will be lonely at home. Return home can reasonably be pursued and attempts made to relieve loneliness by day centre attendance, visiting by volunteers or by admission to residential accommodation at a later stage. The sensation of loneliness does not always correlate with lack of social contacts, however, and some people feel lonely even with many others around them.

Fear of falls is often a major consideration, particularly when an old person has already experienced several falls, perhaps associated with major injury or having lain on the floor for many hours before discovery. When contemplating discharge from hospital it is often useful to ascertain the precise frequency of falls and where they occur. If drop attacks have been experienced while out shopping, for example, this is hardly a reason for not returning home, even if other arrangements have to be made for shopping. Similarly, infrequent falls, with an average of one fall every several months, hardly justify prolonged institutional care. Even where falls are frequent it is often not appreciated by patients and relatives that care in hospital or residential accommodation does not provide protection against falls and their consequences. Indeed, it often happens that the long distances and wide spaces found in hospital and residential homes are more of a hazard than the patient's own home, where the distances are shorter and there is more opportunity for support from walls and furniture. In institutional care, the main advantage is the likelihood that a member of staff will be on hand to help the fallen person up from the floor to prevent complications such as hypothermia. Does this justify permanent institutional care?

The cause of falls should be sought and tackled; it is only with persistent frequent falls or severe loss of confidence as a result of falls that grounds can be justified for an old person not to return home. Indeed, if all the elderly who had falls, or were in danger of falling, were thought to need institutional care, the care system itself would collapse. As it happens, most old people with a tendency to fall express a positive wish to return home and accept the risks of an independent life; these risks are considered a small price to pay for the opportunity to live in their own homes.

As a rule, sympathetic discussion of these factors, with due attention to the anxieties of relatives and friends of the vulnerable old person, allows the situation to be seen in context. While accidents cannot be entirely prevented, it is important for the situation to be seen in perspective by relatives, and for them to realise that the advantages of an independent life for the individual outweigh the risks.

Under times of stress surrounding admission to hospital or discharge, it is tempting to consider solutions which have the short-term advantage of convenience, but which pose major problems over a longer period. This is particularly so when the patient has been recently bereaved, in addition to needing hospital care for other pathology.

Relatives often feel a heavy moral pressure to support elderly people, even when it requires a major social restructuring in the family. One such 'solution' is for an old person to give up her own home to move in with relatives. This type of arrangement provides temporary peace of mind on account of the relief of loneliness and in satisfying a sense of responsibility; help will be at hand if that old person falls and social approval is obtained from other relatives and friends. But it is unfortunately the case that when mixed generations live together there are considerable strains on the family which make it difficult to be emotionally satisfying in the long term to those involved. The short-term gains stem from satisfying a sense of duty and the provision of close supervision, but these are often outweighed by the likelihood of longer-term friction and disruption of relationships. While some few families can live peaceably and even happily together, many find the strains of close living more than they can sustain. Instead of remaining on friendly terms, the relationship between the old person and the younger generation becomes soured and a sequence of unease, strain, hostility and even breakdown occurs. Similar results are seen when the reverse mechanism occurs and the younger generation moves in with the older.

It is sometimes suggested that the Attendance Allowance mentioned earlier is a lubrication which will oil uneasy relationships. While superficially attractive, and of great usefulness where a good and stable support is already available to an old disabled person, the financial inducement of the Attendance Allowance has limitations.

For example, to look after an old person, the relative may have to give up her own income (and the satisfaction of the job), and this financial loss is usually much greater than the Attendance Allowance. In addition to this reduction of income, there may be permanent unemployment after the death of the elderly relative and consequent reduction of the relative's own pension when she retires. Also the very prolonged and close contact between relative and old person means not only a reduced social life for the relative but the danger of the insidious development of a distorted relationship between relative and older person stemming from the great amount of time and the closeness of the interaction they spend together and the lack of other social contacts. In a professional relationship with the disabled elderly there is a distancing between patient and helper which maintains a healthy relationship which may be absent from the close proximity of relative and patient. It may be beneficial for a close relative to find employment outside the home, and for other help to substitute for that relative during working periods. This stype of arrangement is usually successful in preserving the patient/relative relationship even if the relative obtains employment in another caring field.

Another alternative is for the elderly person to be admitted to residential accommodation. For this, an old person usually has to be personally independent in terms of walking or in a wheelchair, continent and without behavioural problems. In point of fact, so many old persons could be considered for admission to residential accommodation that most Social Services departments have long waiting lists or in practice admit emergencies only. Patients in hospital often find that the option of residential accommodation does not exist unless the client is too forgetful, or has a personality problem such that she is too poorly motivated to live at home, or only temporary placement in residential accommodation will be helpful.

In most areas, it is more practical to pursue the possibility of discharge home. Even for the forgetful and poorly motivated it is usually appropriate to consider a trial discharge home as a surprisingly large number of infirm old people manage in their own homes; if discharge home fails, it is necessary to readmit the patient/client to hospital to await a Social Services vacancy.

In general, if a physically disabled person is rational and well motivated, home care with the usual supports is possible. When breakdown occurs, it is usually because such gross physical disability or incontinence has developed that the patient is below the standard for residential accommodation and permanent hospital care has become necessary.

## Setting up a Reasonable Discharge

Concerning most old persons who have problems relating to discharge from hospital it is necessary to counsel the relatives and others involved with the patient to include a discussion of the various alternatives, to talk over anxieties and review possible alternative outcomes.

Return home is the likely outcome on economic and practical grounds. Following discharge it is helpful to monitor the situation and try to avoid over-protectiveness by the relatives, over-dependence by the patient, or both.

All involved with the patient need to know how capable the patient has been while under supervision; good communications between hospital and domiciliary staff may be difficult to set up, but are crucial. With different patients different agencies may provide the crucial follow-up and monitoring system of the patient/client after discharge. Commonly these are the general practitioner through his health visitor or district nurse, or the social worker, and it is necessary to avoid both unnecessary duplication of supervision and the hiatus when each agency leaves it to the other. A day hospital is often an emotionally neutral forum to supervise progress as well as providing the multi-disciplinary team capable of helping a borderline situation. It provides reserve help to cope with many types of problems. If these should be insufficient the patient may be readmitted for a reassessment of the situation in the light of information gained by the discharge.

## Forbidden Phrases

At any stage of the management of an old person with medical problems, there are certain stock phrases which are counter-productive. One of these is: 'He/she should never be left alone.'

It is useful discipline to apply this common instruction to members of one's own family to see how practical it is. To provide supervision of anyone for every hour of every day is beyond the limit of most families and the instruction often meets the emotional needs of the doctor giving the instructions rather than helping.

Does never being alone mean that someone else should be in the same house or even the same room? Does it mean that the companion is not allowed to sleep and possibly miss a call for help? Does it really mean that a companion is not allowed to go out for five minutes, ten minutes or longer? Even in a residential home or hospital, old people may be left unsupervised for hours, so what do such instructions really mean at home?

Another dogmatic statement is: 'He/she will never be able to manage at home again.'. This opinion that an old person will never manage at home alone implies an ability to prognosticate that is usually beyond most doctors' capabilities. No one can really foretell how a person will cope in the future and when such an instruction is given at a time of crisis, illness or bereavement, mistakes are bound to happen. It is better to wait and see how a person fares after the crisis before giving advice; it is a tragedy when a home is surrendered at time of stress and the old person is later unhappy living with relatives or in an institution.

**The 'Jekyll and Hyde' Syndrome**

Earlier we have seen how medical problems may masquerade as social problems; the converse can also occur, and disrupted relationships may be the basic abnormality even though physical disability is the presenting complaint. An example is shown in the following history:

> Mr H aged 74 was referred to hospital when he was bedfast and doubly incontinent; his wife stated that she had to feed, wash and toilet him and that he was capable of no positive activity. Mr H had been in this state for three weeks and over the past six months had become increasingly dependent. Five years previously he had been an in-patient in a psychiatric hospital with a paranoid illness. He was passive and ignored questions about disabilities, but on other topics he was sensible and responsive. He had signs of Parkinsonism with rigidity and akinesia but no tremor. Mr H was admitted to hospital and started on levodopa, reaching a maintenance dose of 4g daily. Within a week he was personally independent on the ward and throughout his stay there was no incontinence. His wife resisted

discharge as she found it hard to believe he was so active, even though his level of activity was demonstrated to her. Eventually he returned home after three weeks in hospital.

Three days later Mr H was referred back to hospital with the information that he was exactly the same on discharge as he had been before admission. He was readmitted and there were no new signs; on the day of readmission he was personally independent and continent and remained so in hospital. This pattern was repeated after a further discharge and Mr H spent a further eighteen days at home before readmission; attempts to find what went wrong at home were unsuccessful. Mr H remained silent on his domestic situation while Mrs H complained bitterly about her husband's disabilities. There seemed little alternative to a further discharge, and day hospital attendance failed to break the resulting impasse; Mrs H became more and more distressed and demanded that her husband be removed from home. A request was made to the local authority for admission to residential accommodation, but the Social Services Department attached no priority to the request since Mr H had a relatively young and healthy wife to care for him. After seven months of complaint Mrs H took an overdose of barbiturates and was admitted to hospital as an attempted suicide. Mr H was admitted to residential accommodation as an emergency and became a permanent resident. He remained happy and active in the residential home while Mrs H returned home after a week in hospital and led her own life apart from her husband.

Ths pattern of events is a recurring one.[11] There is some relatively minor disease which in itself is not sufficient to cause significant disability, but to which problems are attributed; the patient and one relative form the family unit and there is no insight into basic relationship problems; the overt manifestation is of major disability at home, which disappears on admission to hospital and recurs in the domestic setting. The patient is ready for home while in hospital, yet needs hospital care when at home, a combination of circumstances which is guaranteed to produce maximum misunderstanding and friction between domiciliary and hospital workers. We do not yet know the frequency of this sequence of events, and the best ways of dealing with them. Before this syndrome can be diagnosed, complicating illnesses or recurrent adverse drug reactions need to be excluded.

## Conclusion

The problems of the elderly do not fit neatly into administrative divisions between health and social services. If health authorities admit patients whose problems resolve into social problems these in-patients can often ease the work-load on the ward. An elderly person in a hospital ward awaiting a place in residential accommodation is a 'lodger' in the ward, needing little attention and making the work-load of the nursing staff lighter than it would otherwise be; similar arguments apply to day hospital attenders who are awaiting placement in a day centre.

The converse is very different. An old person in residential accommodation who needs hospital care takes a disproportionate amount of time and energy of the residential home staff; similarly at a day centre a client who should really be attending a day hospital takes an unreasonable fraction of the day centre resources. The local authority is therefore at a disadvantage in any misplacement of patient/client. This statement of the situation ignores other factors such as the pace and impetus of a hospital ward, which is slowed by the presence of 'lodgers' awaiting places in residential homes; and, of course, the sick people who may be excluded from hospital treatment by occupation of potential beds by such 'lodgers'.

Many features of the care of the elderly underline the joint responsibilities of health and social services, both at the level of the individual patient/client, and at the planning level. Co-operation and co-ordination are clearly the watchwords if there are to be unified services for the elderly who need help.

## References

1. Pathy, M.S. (1967) 'Clinical Presentation of Myocardial Infarction in the Elderly', *British Heart Journal, 129,* 190-9
2. Burston, G.R., and Moore-Smith, B. (1970) 'Occult Surgical Emergencies in the Elderly', *British Journal of Clinical Practice, 24*, 239-43
3. Morton, E.V.B., and Tyndall, R.M. (1971) 'Physical Illness in 'Social Emergencies' ', *Gerontologia Clinica, 13*, 145-52
4. Williamson, J., Stokoe, I.H., Gray, D., Fisher, M., Smith, A., McGhee, A., and Stephenson, E. (1964) 'Old People at Home: their Unreported Needs', *Lancet, i*, 1117-20
5. Brocklehurst, J.C., Carty, M.H., Leeming, J.T., and Robinson, J.M. (1978) 'Medical Screening of Old People Accepted for Residential Care', *Lancet, ii*, 141-3
6. Carter, K., and Evans, T.N. (1978) *Intentions and Achievements in Admissions of the Elderly to Residential Care*, Clearing House for Local Authority Social

Services Research, No. 9, pp. 71-99
7. Smith, R.S., and Lowther, C.P. (1976) 'Follow-up Study of Two Hundred Admissions to a Residential Home', *Age and Ageing, 5*, 176-80
8. Mechanic, D. (1966) 'Response Factors in Illness: the Study of Illness Behaviour', *Social Psychiatry, 1*, 11-20
9. Lowther, C.P., and Williamson, J. (1966) 'Old People and their Relatives', *Lancet, ii*, 1459-60
10. Isaacs, B. (1971) 'Geriatric Patients: do their Families care?' *British Medical Journal, 4,* 282-6
11. Boyd, R.V., and Woodman, J. (1978) 'The Jekyll-and-Hyde Syndrome', *Lancet, ii*, 671-2

# 10 THE FRAIL ELDERLY – A SOCIAL WORKER'S PERSPECTIVE

Olive Stevenson

This chapter is written at a time of general gloom and anxiety about the effects of present British government policies upon health and social services. Indeed this is reinforced both in the United Kingdom and other Western nations by the current economic situations. In these contexts, the care of the frail elderly stands out as of major concern. First, because the well known predictions about numbers, well outlined in the discussion document *A Happier Old Age,*[1] made it clear that not restraint but considerable growth in the health and social care sector was essential if we were even to stay where we were. Second, until now the frail elderly have not been a group to 'ask for more'. Many who have seen harder times will say that they 'manage quite well, thank you'. Whilst one may respect the independence and resilience that such comments indicate, they also show that some are not aware of what could be done to make their lives more comfortable and more enjoyable, whether this be related to their environmental, bodily, mental or spiritual well-being.

A recent comprehensive study of poverty in the United Kingdom[2] shows that the elderly (together with large families) suffer the greatest relative poverty in our society, even taking the most conservative and widely accepted indices. It is no comfort to them that new pension schemes will benefit the elderly by the end of the century and statements by the present government indicate that schemes of linking such pensions to the cost of living cannot be taken for granted in the future. Furthermore, for the frail elderly, it is misleading to consider poverty solely in terms of direct financial provision. A wide variety of services are needed for some to make life tolerable, leave alone enjoyable. Whilst it may be true that if one is rich enough one can 'buy in' many services, the vast majority of the frail elderly will continue to depend on services which are, at least in part, subsidised (home helps are the obvious example). What is more, organised provision is integral to good social care. Money alone is useless, for example, if there are insufficient chiropodists in the area to provide the service. This is obvious. Yet its implications deserve examination, for, whatever its merits, our system of local government, reinforced by the stated policy of 'non-interference' by the present government, creates, even fosters, territorial injustice on a scale which would make it prudent for every old person to have a Consumer's Guide before deciding where to live in retirement.

In the face of massive, and increasing, deficiencies in social care provision, it would be easy to say that social work is an expendable luxury. What we need are more home helps, day care, short-term admission to residential care, incontinence laundry services . . . the list is endless. If doctors were asked to rank these in order of priority, one suspects that social work would come very near the bottom.

## The Social Work Task with and for Elderly Clients

The purpose of this chapter is not to seek to push social work up that ladder of priorities, but to analyse some aspects of what social work can and should contribute, within the overall context of health and social care, the integration of which is essential for the individual well-being of the frail elderly.

Amongst the images of social workers held by others, notably doctors, two can be picked out. The first is that their function is to mobilise resources, home helps for example. The second, less common perhaps, but still noised abroad, is that social workers do something called 'casework', which is a bit like psychotherapy, but not so 'deep' and is intended to help people with their emotional problems. There is considerable scepticism about its efficacy and a slight aura of mystery surrounds the process. I shall pursue the implications of these 'images' later.

There is now evidence that most social workers spend most of their time not in face-to-face contact with the client but in doing things for and about the client. This is certainly true of social workers in hospitals and in Social Services departments. It is also generally agreed that Social Services departments have allocated their less experienced and less qualified workers to the care of the frail elderly.[4] They are often dealt with by social work assistants. Few social workers defend this as the ideal arrangement; they explain it as a reaction to the pressure of other demands upon a service still not fully qualified professionally; other cases, notably those involving non-accidental injury to children, they argue, have had to take priority. However, even in authorities with a very high proportion of qualified staff,* work with the frail elderly

*It should be noted that the percentage of qualified social work staff in Social Services departments varies from (approximately) 10 to 90 per cent – another example of territorial injustice.

has not commanded the same interest and enthusiasm as some other aspects of social work.[5] This may simply be part of a wider problem concerning social and professional attitudes to the elderly, in which social workers do not differ from, *inter alia*, the medical profession. There are signs that the tide might be on the turn so far as social work is concerned. But, writing now, it is difficult to predict whether, in the next decade or so, the will will be there to provide a social work service of quality, if the way – in terms of resources, organisational structures and post-qualifying training – can be found. Whatever the future, at present we have the oddity that the elderly command the lion's share of social service budgets but the mouse's share of qualified social workers' time.

Let me now refer to the popular images of social work. The fact that social workers spend a great deal of time with people who are not the client does not in my view diminish their claim to certain skills. Skill does not lie only in a direct transaction between patient/client and the worker. Although other professionals must also undertake these activities (and might do well to consider how effectively they do so), it is arguable that social workers should spend most time at the 'interface' between various people whose services the clients need and that, if they are skilled enough, they effect smoother communication and co-operation to the benefit of the client. (Of course, there are bad social workers. I am writing of what might be and sometimes is.)

The frail elderly frequently require a wide variety of services if they are to remain in the community. It is, in my view, appropriate for the social worker to act as mobiliser and co-ordinator of these services. What is the knowledge and skill required? In part, it is practical administrative 'know-how', and this should not be denigrated, given our complex societal web. In part, it is the use of creative, imaginative abilities, attempting to solve the apparently insoluble. Given the absolute shortage of resources we face, this capacity to 'think of another way' is likely to assume great significance. Mobilising resources is not a simple matter of making phone calls and writing letters. It involves flexible responses to individual problems and needs. But there is a third and crucial component of social work skill in this respect, perhaps the one which distinguishes it from administrative competence and resourcefulness: that is, continuous appraisal, before and during the arranging of services, of the effects this may have on the elderly person him or herself. What does he/she really want? How are suggestions to be presented? How is rejection of certain kinds of help to be dealt with – the hurt feelings of neighbours, for example? In other words, at the centre of the social worker's remit, whatever he is doing *about* people, he must be doing it *with* them at the same time. He must do this for two reasons. First, morally, there is an obligation to respect, in so far as is possible, the wishes of the person, who is an individual with a right to the maximum degree of independence in decision-making. Second, plans which ignore the wishes of the individuals concerned are usually defeated! Thus there is a sense in which the two images of social work which I described earlier come together. The practical activity on behalf of clients is integral to the social work task; yet the need to formulate the plans with the person concerned and, in so doing, to relate sensitively to the feelings of others (relatives, volunteers, etc.) is crucial and will often involve the discussion of delicate areas with all concerned.

This is the stuff of any social work. It is not just to do with the frail elderly. Until recently, social work education and training, as reflected in the literature, have not effected a successful integration between those aspects of the task described, somewhat disparagingly, as 'practical' and those which describe processes of psychosocial adjustments of individuals and families. In the last five years or so, however, due in part to the influence of certain writers from the USA[6,7] and the espousal of their ideas by some British educators and practitioners,[8] attempts have been made to look at the task of the social worker with a new perspective derived from systems theory and described, somewhat pompously, as 'the unitary approach'. Briefly, this approach encourages the social worker to identify the 'targets for change' and to work towards constructive intervention in whatever aspect of the client's life it is felt to be most urgent and profitable. This is not the place to discuss the merits of the approach. But it offers an opportunity to break away from a meaningless dichotomy between 'material' and 'emotional' help. It is part of the skill of the social worker to decide with the client (and this may take time) what they both regard as the most important focus for their efforts to effect change. For example, the processes by which an elderly woman is helped to decide whether or not she will enter residential care – a practical decision at one level – may be inextricably linked to her reactions to a relatively recent bereavement. An understanding of these reactions, now fairly well established in the literature,[9] helps the worker to respond more perceptively to the client. It also helps him to help others to understand who are involved in the decision and who may become irritated by the elderly person's vacillations. Another welcome trend in social work literature, following some useful research into 'consumer reactions',[10,11] is the emphasis upon clarification of the purpose of the exchange between client and worker.

Although it has not been specifically applied to work with the elderly, it is easy to see how important it is for an elderly person to understand what 'the man from the welfare' has to offer or wants to find out. In historical terms, the welfare role is a very new one, as compared, for example, with that of the doctor. (Although, in fairness, some might suggest that the medical profession, too, could on occasion with profit clarify the purpose of their questions or comments!)

Thus far, it has been argued that the essence of social work lies in a mixture of practical activity, often involving contact with others, with support or intervention in relation to psychosocial problems. The skill lies in getting the mixture right for particular individuals and situations.

## Social Work and Interprofessional Co-operation

Another aspect of social work activity likely to be of particular interest to the medical profession concerns the necessity of co-operation and collaboration between the two professions. The issue is not contentious, but the means to achieve it are. What are the structures, especially those at local level, most likely to achieve it? There has been something which may crudely be described as a 'post-Seebohm reaction',* with cries for a return to social work specialisation by client groups, of whom the elderly would be one. It is interesting to note that the BMA,[12] giving evidence to the Seebohm Committee, deplored the fragmentation of social work service at that time.

> The present fragmentation has caused inco-ordination of activity in the field and consequent duplication of effort and risk of conflicting advice being offered, especially where departmental policies vary. This leads to confusion on both the part of the general practitoner and the public, who are often unsure to whom to refer patients or to whom to turn for advice. At present the selection of client and caseworker is often more by chance than design owing to the imprecise nature of the work and a lack of overall guidance. An all purpose social selfare service could act as a clearing house in this

*The Seebohm Committee (F. Seebohm, *Report of The Committee on Local Authority and Allied Personal Social Services*, Cmnd. 3703 (HMSO, London, 1968)) examined the structure of local government personal social services and recommended a unified service. The precise interpretation of their recommendations has been varied but all personal social services are provided within the local authority by one Social Services Department.

> respect and refer cases to the appropriate social worker. This would also provide a better career structure. There is too high a degree of specialisation early on in the social worker's career with consequent isolation of groups of social workers according to departmental aims. Furthermore, the development of numerous specialities encourages differentiation in title, status and salary scale and this, in turn, causes dissatisfaction among staff who essentially undertake duties of a similar nature contributing to the general welfare of the family (p. 159, para. 510).

A certain rosiness has clouded the spectacles of those who look back upon 'pre-Seebohm' days. There is no evidence to support the view that *in general* the quality of social work service has deteriorated since then (which is not to say that this has not happened in some localities).

However that may be, it is no excuse for failing critically to examine the present quality of social work service and, in particular, the arrangements which need to be made to ensure maximum co-operation between the professions. This has complex implications for specialisation in social work in Social Services departments. It is not self-evident, as some doctors seem to think, that attachment to the medical centre, be it hospital or health centre, is inevitably the best arrangement. It is not clear whether specialisation should be in terms of conventional client groupings, 'the elderly', or whether multi-disciplinary specialist community terms are the right way forward. These issues are explored in a forthcoming book.[13] For this purpose, it suffices to say that a number of variables have to be taken into account in determining patterns of specialisation. One can identify at least six:

(1) the need for particular expertise in individual workers (analogous to the medical specialist);
(2) the value ascribed to generic service to a given geographical area by the same individuals (which, *inter alia*, may encourage community development and participation);
(3) the arrangements made for work to be organised inside a team more efficiently for the benefit of clients ('intake teams' are an example);
(4) the need for certain specialisms to be developed, either to promote a significant field of service (such as the finding of adoptive and foster homes) or because of the special skills required (such as work with the deaf);
(5) the allowance to be made for staff to develop special interests;

(6) the need for arrangements to facilitate co-operation and collaboration with other occupational groups (of whom doctors are only one; teachers and supplementary benefits officials are two other examples).

That the last of these should perhaps be given highest priority in relation to the frail elderly is a view with which I would have much sympathy, given the interaction of medical and social problems. But one must acknowledge the complexities of the debate because those who manage social services have to balance these variables in determining patterns of specialisation. Nor does the emergence of new forms of specialisation mark the end of generic training and initial 'general practice'. Few would wish to train social workers again to begin as specialists, any more than it is considered appropriate in medicine.

Behind organisational structures lie other, equally important, questions which affect interprofessional communication; questions which include problems of role, status, educational and social backgrounds, all of which affect the perceptions which different occupational groups have of each other. These issues have been explored by myself and a colleague in relation to child abuse.[14] This has been a particularly sensitive area, in which the anxieties of all occupational groups involved have played a part in stimulating new efforts towards more effective communication. The fundamental issues, however, are no different in relation to professional co-operation concering the frail elderly. It is quite possible that a 'granny' tragedy similar to the Maria Colwell inquiry[15] will before long focus attention and maybe criticism on this area of interprofessional work. Although all occupational groups have a responsibility in this matter, social workers have a crucial role in facilitating interprofessional communication.

Many other aspects of social work with the frail elderly could be discussed; only a selection of key issues follow.

## Residential Care

The first concerns residential care. When one considers the vulnerability of the frail elderly to various forms of exploitation or maltreatment and the difficulties of finding staff of suitable calibre to care for them, a problem common to hospitals and homes, one can perhaps give half a cheer that the present cuts in public expenditure make it inevitable that only a fraction of the people, for whom some would argue residential care is needed, will be offered it. But it can only be half a cheer, for the community care problems are daunting. In any case, concern remains about the homes which we have and the quality of life which they provide for the residents. As with care of the mentally handicapped, though perhaps less vociferous, there has been a somewhat contentious debate about the appropriate qualification for those who run old people's homes. Many 'officers-in-charge' are not qualified. Of those who are, nursing has been the traditional qualification. As part of a wider debate about the status of, and qualities required in, residential staff, the Central Council for Education and Training in Social Work issued a discussion document in 1973.[16] This made certain assumptions, generally accepted in social work at the time, that the appropriate training for the leadership of residential establishments (prisons and hospitals excepted) was social work. Training policies developed from that have not been seriously challenged, although the development of new schemes for in-service training leading to 'a Certificate of Social Service', which can be taken, *inter alia*, by those possessing nursing qualifications, has somewhat muddied the policy waters. The figures of residential staff with any training, leave alone a social work qualification, remain very low, although substantial progress has been made.*

The suggestion that social work rather than nursing is the appropriate qualification does not, of course, imply that the many nurses, presently 'officers-in-charge', are not doing admirable and dedicated work. The issue is what the nature of the residential task really is and therefore what training for it is appropriate.[18] Nor is it altogether clear whether effective 'generic' arguments can be advanced for residential social work training in the same terms as for field social workers. For example, the growing numbers of the very frail, who, in other circumstances might have been admitted to geriatric hospitals, suggest there is a need, possibly growing, for nursing as well as social work in old people's homes. But there is now a recognition that residential staff need to be aware of ways in which the quality of life, emotional and intellectual, can be enhanced and that the desired model, to borrow a phrase from a study of residential care for the physically handicapped,[19] is more of 'horticulture than warehousing'. (However, the authors of this study point out that the 'horticultural model', seemingly more attractive, has its dangers if it defines success solely in terms of growth or improvement.) In any case, whether social workers do this

*Of all students completing Certificate of Qualification in Social Work courses in 1977, 2.9 per cent went into residential work. The percentage rose to 6.3 in 1978.[17]

better than other occupational groups will probably remain contentious. But the social work profession (through the British Association of Social Workers) has accepted a responsibility for residential work across a wide spectrum of provision, including elderly persons' homes. It is an onerous task and the implications are far-reaching.

However, the proportion of old people in any form of residential care remains relatively small. Certainly there is no evidence of a general breakdown of a sense of responsibility for elderly relatives. Some professionals, especially geriatricians, nurses and residential care staff, see the most tragic rejections. But to infer from this a general breakdown in filial duty is quite misleading. What is clear, however, is that geographical mobility and housing problems create serious difficulties for caring relatives.

## Support for 'The Carers'

These facts are well known to the medical profession and need not be elaborated. What urgently needs attention, however, are the implications for support of the 'community carers'. Social work is only part of such community care and it is no part of my argument to give it a significance out of proportion to the rest. Since social work service to the elderly is deficient anyway, the efforts which are made by social workers are usually directed to those living alone or with a spouse. That is understandable, given present problems. However, it is regrettable that so little social work support is being given to those who care in their own homes for the frail elderly. We have little empirical evidence to test in what ways, if at all, family and neighbourhood breakdowns in community care can be averted. Common sense suggests that practical relief of one kind or another from the daily, unremitting strain, especially where dementia is involved, will be valuable. But there has been little exploration of emotional rèlief, of the possible gains from expression and discussion of feelings of anger and of guilt, for example. Social workers who have devoted time and training to family therapy, which explores just such situations, have rarely undertaken this work with an old person as the identified problem, although the conceptual framework is very similar for the treatment process, in which, for example, an adolescent is the identified 'patient'. Such work with families caring for the elderly is complicated by the fact that the adult child has memories, conscious and unconscious, of how he was treated by the now dependent adult; furthermore, the ego restraints in the elderly are loosened and he in turn will be reviving memories of his treatment as a child, sometimes confused with how he perceives his position in the present role reversal.

We have little scientific proof that intervention into such areas of family dynamics is profitable. It is notoriously difficult in this area to devise experiments which will control variables to demonstrate outcomes. But this chapter is not about the problems of such research. We all operate on certain assumptions until proven wrong. The assumption here is that we cannot afford to ignore the intense dynamics created in some families caring for their frail elderly. Morally, they are 'our neighbours' and they need help. Professionally, one may hypothesise that, for some, relief of emotional tensions may avert tragedy; for example, the breakdown in the health of the carers, the abuse of the elderly or reception into long-stay care. 'Relief of emotional tension' is a complex phrase: it may just mean 'letting off steam', but the intervention may be at a much subtler level, concerned with an exploration of the feelings created by the situation. It is, therefore, not 'anybody's job', though no doubt different people play different parts at different times. One of the social worker's skills and tasks is to identify and reinforce who does what for whom in ensuring this essential relief of tension.

In the context of home care a social trend which cannot be ignored is that of the increased number of women going out to work. It has been pointed out that in the age band 35-54, the economic activity rates for married women have risen from 25 per cent in 1951 to 62 per cent in the last general household survey.[20] Such figures would be much higher if we had accurate figures of women in part-time and casual employment. These facts may be linked to the evidence of growing and persistent unemployment in certain sectors of the male population; the implications for changing sex roles within the family are clear. Whatever our social or moral views (or prejudices) may be about such trends, there is little likelihood of reversing them. More and more families depend upon two incomes and there is evidence of the psychological value of work outside the home for some unsupported women.[21] These trends pose problems in social policy for the care of the frail elderly which go far beyond the particular question of the role of the social worker. But, in practical terms, it means that many social workers, in their daily activities on behalf of the frail elderly, will have to look outside the family and seek to mobilise other resources for the environmental support needed. There will also be casework skills involved in helping some men with their feelings about the role reversal consequent upon our present economic problems. Early retirement and redundancy for some men, whilst their wives continue in employment, will place upon them a greater share of responsibility for the support of elderly relatives than they bargained for!

Another aspect of the social worker's role (rarely developed) concerns the possibility of improving the quality of relationships which exist between the frail elderly and those relatives with whom they do not live, who are concerned and caring but with whom relationships have become tense or ambivalent. Such work has been accepted for many years as integral to child welfare. Social workers involved with children separated from their parents have, since 1948, accepted it as essential to good professional practice to seek to maintain and strengthen these links even where those children were unlikely ever to live at home. In the course of such work, delicate and sensitive areas of feelings had to be explored on both sides. (And practical things had to be done too, for example, about transport.) We demean the frail elderly if we ignore the tensions and interactional problems which exist in all relationships but which may, on occasions, for a variety of reasons get worse as the years go by. This may be in part because in the process of ageing the elderly person may become more self-centred, more demanding and more dependent; or it may be because of family difficulties unrelated to the old person in question.

## The Changing Structure of the Family

An additional dimension to this inter-generational stress is that related to the trends concerning divorce and remarriage. Between 1951 and 1976, the number of divorces had risen from 31,000 to 36,000 and the rate per 1,000 of the married population has risen from 2 to 10. Over 60 per cent of divorcing couples have children under 16. Remarriage is also very popular. In 1976, nearly one-third of all marriages were remarriages for one or both partners.[22] And divorce rates amongst remarried couples are much higher than for those married once only. Hundreds of thousands of older people are going to have to make relationships with new partners of their children. Sometimes this may offer opportunities to start afresh without the problems surrounding earlier years when 'in-law' tensions were at their height. Sometimes it may mean that the decision to offer an elderly new parent-in-law a home or close support is made from newly found respect and affection and not only from a sense of duty. But, for many elderly people, the time in their lives when stability and continuity are assuming greater significance will be the very time when they are confronted with the complexities of changed relationships with former sons and daughters-in-law of whom they may have become fond. And, for some, the critical time for them to decide where and with whom to live or live near will be the time when a reconstituted family is seeking to find a new equilibrium. This new family may include children and teenagers who have grown up thinking of their grandparents as fixed points in the universe. They may suddenly find new people presented as grandparents and experience difficulties, the nature of which they do not fully understand, with 'long-time' grandparents, borne of the tensions which have arisen between adults. Obviously, as with so many aspects of changing family patterns, not only do people overcome such difficulties with generosity and with love but some of the newly formed bonds may be strong and good. We would be quite unrealistic, however, if we did not take account of such widespread events in modern family life and of the way in which they impinge upon the support which older people receive. For example, when things go wrong in our relationships, it is quite common to hide them from our parents for as long as possible. The phrase 'I don't want to worry them' is a part truth; there is another layer that feels guilty and fears reproach. A younger generation, even of adults, often underestimates the capacity of older people to forgive and to accept. Perhaps childhood fears and anxieties linger on in us and inhibit communications, even between the middle-aged and their parents.

Many of those who experience the break-up of their children's marriages will be 'the young elderly' and not the group of frail elderly with whom this essay is primarily concerned. None the less, the trend is relevant to my theme. The general effects upon families of this shifting membership need our close attention and the elderly are included in this. It has been suggested[23] that we should give up the term 'nuclear family' and talk instead of the 'modified extended family' as representing more realistically the situation in our society today. Greater geographical mobility, although highly variable between areas, is a fact. There is no evidence to suggest that kinship networks have broken down in an emotional sense. Therefore, the ways in which elderly persons help and are helped at points when their children's marriages break or are remade may have a direct relevance to the way they feel and others feel about them at a later stage when they are less self-reliant.

Much of 'this family business', with all its attendant stress and strain, will be handled privately. There will not (and perhaps should not) be a place for social workers. But, even at present through court cases matters of access and custody of children, social workers are involved. It is interesting to note that the role of grandparents in such cases is now being raised, even to the point of legislating for grandparents to apply to the courts for access to their grandchildren when one or both parents have died. Thus it is not fanciful to suggest that if social workers were to think more positively about the wider family in help offered and plans made at such times, there might be benefits for all three generations.

Whilst there is no evidence of significant breakdown in relationships between aged parents and their children, there is evidence of a major problem in that so many elderly people have no children or have outlived them, and that where there are children, they are few in number. In one sample in three areas of England,[24] it was found that:

> Today's survivors from the 19th century were far from fecund even by today's standards: 30% were completely childless and another 45% had only one or two children. The averages of child bearing show that as a group they fell short of reproducing themselves . . . (Of women living alone over 75) . . . nearly 40% were childless and another 23% had only one child. In all respects . . . the composition of the [this] population in the next decade will be very similar to that of today (p. 18).

This study further examines the issue of spatial proximity to their parents of those who have children. Although there will be wide regional variations it is concluded that it is likely that of those who have children 'at least half will be living within six miles of their nearest offspring' (p. 23).

Thus many of the frail elderly about whom social workers will be most concerned will have little by way of practical support from their own younger kith and kin, either because they simply do not exist or because they live too far away. This relates to the earlier point concerning the role of the social worker in locating, mobilising, co-ordinating and even creating community support, a task far more complex and skilled than is sometimes recognised. But it also raises two central questions with which the social worker must be concerned, risk and dependency.

**Risk and Dependency**

Many old people live on their own or with elderly spouses and the phrase 'at risk' is frequently heard. There are complex issues involved in this notion. First, there is the question – what kind of risk are we talking about – physical or psychological? Both are involved and they are, to an extent, interrelated. Second, there is the question, who is worrying about 'risk' – the elderly person, those responsible for direct care, those responsible for indirect care, or, a vaguer but none the less significant group, the wider community? Third, any discussion of risk is inseparable from the general question of the balance between dependence and independence which is crucial throughout our lives and which shifts, subtly and in different degrees and ways, in old age. We are sometimes exhorted to let the old 'live dangerously'. This is an over-simplified statement which requires examination both from the point of view of those who are old and those who care for them.

This chapter, focused upon social work, only touches upon a major issue of preventable accidents both inside and outside the home, whose cost to the Health Service is vast and which frequently set the frail elderly on the road to decline. 'Living dangerously' is acceptable only when the danger is a reflection of normal everyday life in a reasonably safe environment. Many of our frail elderly people live in homes with unnecessary hazards. Whilst it is not a social worker's responsibility to tack down the stair carpet, it is (along with others) to observe acutely and to see what can be done to make a home safer. Similarly, an organised response to hazards outside the home (for example in relation to transport services) is *in part* a responsibility of the profession, in conjunction with others. Transport is particularly important in combating isolation and maintaining a degree of independence.

Another aspect of risk with which social workers are often concerned is 'self-neglect'. There are a few rather dramatic cases, in which an old person says in effect, 'I want none of you,' and proceeds to live an eccentric, idiosyncratic life, often involving neglect of basic hygiene. Here the problem is more often what the local community and the professionals can tolerate than what the old person is feeling. One cannot ignore the feelings of neighbours, especially if they are disturbed practically and emotionally, by the old person's eccentricity; but most social workers would be extremely reluctant to invoke the law enabling the person to be removed from home, preferring to seek compromises, such as occasional cleaning-up procedures.

Although such cases cause a stir, far more common and in a sense more worrying are those where self-neglect gradually becomes apparent which, unchecked, may lead to serious physical problems. This neglect centres upon heating, eating and hygiene. Social workers have always to walk the tightrope between allegations of interference, and of neglecting their duty to protect the vulnerable. This aspect of their work, which is sometimes called 'surveillance', gives rise to many professional dilemmas and criticism from outside. It may involve 'checking' (for example, whether there is food in the larder) which goes beyond what is normally acceptable and it certainly involves detailed questions which require responses more precise than 'Oh yes, dear, I manage to keep warm.' Many of the older generation know relatively little about basic nutrition and health care – a lesson for the future but a problem for the present. If one adds to this the mild but chronic depression which is common in the frail elderly, there seems little doubt that there is a role for social work in the assessment and surveillance of this kind of risk. I cannot accept that this is intrusive: it is surely part of a compassionate service to those many frail elderly people who have no children or near relatives to do it for them. One of the issues with which we are currently preoccupied, however, is how far, in a time of scarce resources and qualified staff, assistants, home helps and volunteers can be trained to spot risk or to report to qualified workers in such a way that risk can be inferred from the report.

However, physical risk has to be related to psychological attitudes, especially anxiety. This is an issue which puzzles me. Was the image of serene old age always a myth? Or is it related to the fact that the old today are required to adapt more often and more dramatically than in days gone by? Whatever the answer, there is no doubt that the anxiety level of the elderly person is a powerful factor in determining the extent to which he or she will 'go adventuring'. Social workers have to work with old people to decide to what extent certain physical risk taking is crucial to their psychological well-being. This is a highly individual matter. The recent example of the octogenarian who enjoys trips in hovercraft, helicopters and down the mines is exceptional. For her, the risk is well worth it. The task for the carers, be they directly involved as relatives or residential staff, or indirectly, as field social workers, is to work out, for a given individual, what is so important to his sense of personal autonomy and integrity that the risk is justified, even essential. Thus it is not helpful to make global statements about 'living dangerously'. We have to be more precise in our formulations for individuals.

Social workers have also to address the question – 'who is worried?'

Furthermore, these anxieties can become collusive between the carers and the elderly person, each of whom imputes the anxiety to the other. We can disentangle two different strands. One is related to love, anger and guilt; the other to accountability. That is to say, one is concerned with ourselves as people, both personally and professionally, with past and present experiences and feelings influencing our attitudes to the elderly (our own relatives and, by projection, other people's). The other is concerned with organisational roles and what is expected of social workers (and other professionals) in protection of the vulnerable. Both operate powerfully in relation to the care of the elderly, but social workers have had the latter strongly reinforced by the many inquiries into non-accidental injury resulting in the deaths of children.

Regarding the first issue, it has been implicit in this argument that it is part of the role of the social worker to seek to help those who care for elderly persons with the feelings which give rise to excessive anxiety about risk-taking. This must involve a measure of personal insight in the professional. To discuss the apparent need to wrap granny in cotton wool – the reasons for wanting to do so and the dangers in so doing – this is the essence of social work. There is no easy answer to the second problem, especially when neighbours and friends are pressing for action to be taken because the strain upon them (for example) of a mentally confused old person is felt to be intolerable. Whilst one would explore every avenue of support, there must come a time when residential care is necessary because those most directly involved cannot bear the anxiety any longer. This cannot always coincide with the old person's wishes and, like so much in social work, painful choices may have to be made in situations of conflict. Neither the elderly person nor those who are involved are *de facto* 'right' in what they want.

Such observations lead inevitably to questions about the power of the social worker. Individual social workers, faced with a grave shortage of resources, often feel powerless whilst being regarded by clients (and perhaps sometimes by other professionals) as being powerful because they represent Social Services departments which control resources. Whilst in practical terms the field level social worker at times may have very little to offer, it would be wrong to equate power simply with available resources. Those who educate social workers recognise that simply advising is a form of influence, and hence power. Some people are vulnerable to pressure concerning those choices open to them, of which the most important is usually the decision to enter residential care. Responsibility for helping the frail elderly reach such decisions is a heavy ethical professional burden. At the centre of good practice must be an assessment, worked out with the client, of what is right for him, a person with rights, needs and responsibilities like all the rest of us. It is in this personal interaction that the skill of much social work lies.

In writing this chapter, I have been aware throughout that the current practice falls far short of what has been suggested as the appropriate role for social workers with the elderly. But without an ideal, there can be no progress.

## Acknowledgement

The author would like to acknowledge a particular debt to Cherry Rowlings, Senior Research Fellow at Keele University, who has shared in much of the thinking and discussion that has led to this chapter.

## References

1. DHSS (1978) *A Happier Old Age*, HMSO, London
2. Townsend, P. (1979) *Poverty in the United Kingdom*, Penguin, Harmondsworth
3. See, for example, Goldberg, E.M., and Fruin, D.J. (1976) 'Towards Accountability in Social Work', *BJSW* (Spring), *6* 1, 10
4. DHSS (Social Work Research Project) (1978) *Social Service Teams: the Practitioner's View*, HMSO, London
5. Ibid.
6. Pincus, A., and Minahan, A. (1973) *Social Work Practice: Model and Method*, Peacock, Itasca, Illinois
7. Goldstein, H.A. (1973) *Unitary Approach*, University of South Carolina Press, Columbia, South Carolina
8. For example, Specht, H., and Vickery, A. (1977) *Integrating Social Work Methods*, National Institute Social Services Library No. 31, George Allen and Unwin, London
9. See, for example, Murray Parkes, C. (1972) *Bereavement*, Tavistock Publications, London
10. Sainsbury, E. (1975) *Social Work with Families*, Routledge and Kegan Paul, London
11. Mayer, J.E., and Timms, N. (1970) *The Client Speaks*, Routledge and Kegan Paul, London
12. Cmnd 3703 (Seebohm Report) (1968) *Report of the Committee on Local Authority and Allied Personal Social Services*, HMSO, London
13. Stevenson, O. (in preparation) *Specialisation in Social Work*, George Allen and Unwin, London
14. Hallet, C., and Stevenson, O. (1980) *Child Abuse: Aspects of Interprofessional Co-operation*, George Allen and Unwin, London
15. DHSS (1974) *Report of the Committee of Inquiry into the Care and Supervision Provided in Relation to Maria Colwell*, HMSO, London
16. Central Council for Education and Training in Social Work (CCETSW) (1973) *Residential Work is Part of Social Work*, CCETSW, London

17. CCETSW (1979) *Abstracts of Data 1978*, CCETSW, London
18. Currently a project at Keele University in conjunction with Cheshire Social Services Department is examining this issue.
19. Miller, E.J., and Gwynne, G.V. (1972) *A Life Apart*, Tavistock Publications, London
20. Parker, R.A. (1978) 'Foster Care in Context', *Adoption and Fostering, 93*, 3, 27-32
21. Brown, G.W., and Harris, T. (1978) *Social Origins of Depression,* Tavistock Publications, London
22. CSO (1979) *Social Trends*, HMSO, London
23. Morgan, D.H.J. (1975) *Social Theory and the Family*, Routledge and Kegan Paul, London
24. Abrams, M. (1978) *Beyond Three Score Years and Ten*, Age Concern, Mitcham, Surrey

# 11 INSTITUTIONAL CARE

J. Grimley Evans

The emphasis in planning provision for medical and social services for the elderly over the last two decades has been on the prevention of institutionalisation. This policy has been reflected in the expansion of home help and other domiciliary services, provision of day hospitals and day centres and an increasing commitment among hospital geriatric services to out-patient and community work. Despite this intensive activity the three censuses in 1951, 1961 and 1971 show that institutionalisation rates among the very elderly (aged 80 and over) have been increasing steeply.[1] The increase has been mostly in residential homes, and although short-term elective admissions to residential homes have recently become more common, most of the increase from 1951 to 1971 in the proportion of elderly people in residential care will reflect permanent institutionalisation. The increase is not attributable in any important degree to changes in the age structure of the open-ended age grouping of 80 years and over. Nor is it attributable to a recent policy of admitting less necessary cases; indeed what evidence there is suggests that elderly people entering residential care now are more disabled physically and mentally than their predecessors of ten or twenty years ago.[2,3]

This finding does not necessary imply that the policy of community care has been misconceived or has failed. There is abundant evidence that the main support for the elderly in preventing institutionalisation comes from the family rather than from the state, and there is equally abundant evidence that the amount of family support available to the elderly has been declining over the last twenty years and is to decline yet further in the future. Townsend[4] found evidence that the probability of an elderly person having to apply for placement in residential care was inversely related to the number of his or her surviving children. Unfortunately, owing to the decline in mean family size over the first forty years of this century, the average number of potentially dutiful children available to parents has fallen by about 20 per cent since the start of the National Health Service and will decline by a further 20 per cent before the end of the century.[1] This effect will be offset to some degree by increasing marriage rates during this century; the proportion of never-married women aged 65 and over in 1951 was 16.2

per cent compared with 14.7 per cent in 1971 and a projected 9.3 per cent in 1991. Even without the concomitant increase in divorce which may disrupt patterns of family support even when remarriage has occurred, the number of children available per 100 women aged 65 and over will have fallen from 210 in 1951 to 145 in 1991. Adding to this the increasing migration of children away from the family home and the high rates of employment among married women[5,6] who have traditionally borne the main responsibility for caring for aged relatives, it is scarcely surprising that the demand on statutory institutional care has been rising. The effect of unavailability of family support in increasing demand for chronic care will be obvious enough, but it is less widely appreciated that the need for acute hospital care will also be increased. Without immediately available family support, an attack of influenza or other minor illness may necessitate the admission of an old person to hospital for nursing care.

More optimistic views on the future needs of the elderly population for institutional care have been urged.[7] These views depend heavily on Scottish studies suggesting that many old people in residential care could manage in sheltered housing, were this available. In Scotland the provision of hospital beds is much more generous than in England and Wales, so the situation there is unlikely to represent the plight of the rest of the United Kingdom.

It is important to emphasise that there is little evidence that families are feeling less obligation to contribute to the support of their elderly relatives than was once the case. Where family support is available, it is usually given and in quantitative terms is a far greater contribution to the support of elderly people than are the statutory domiciliary services.[8] This should be stated loudly and consistently, for if it became widely thought that the current fashion is for families to neglect their elderly, such a fashion would undoubtedly be created.

A number of other factors may be invoked to explain why the increasing pressure towards institutionalisation has had particular effect on residential care. One of these factors is the increasing awareness of resource limitation leading to the consideration of relative priorities among applicants for residential care. Wise husbandry demands that no one should be allowed into residential care who can be supported at a lower degree of dependency. For this reason co-operation between Social Services departments and geriatric services has led in several centres around the country to routine medical screening of applicants for residential care to ensure that no remediable medical condition is contributing to the applicant's inability to cope in the community.[9]

There is no statutory requirement for medical involvement in the placement of an old person in a residential home and this co-operation between social services and geriatric departments represents one of the ways in which local initiative and goodwill are necessary to compensate for deficiencies in statutory arrangements. A second reason why the increase in institutionalisation has fallen almost exclusively on residential care is a change in hospital practice over the last two decades, so that many people who might have found a permanent place in hospital in 1951 will not be able to do so today. These changes in non-psychiatric hospital function are to be examined in more detail below, but there is also evidence of changes in psychiatric hospital practice. Shulman and Arie[10] have drawn attention to the fall in admission rates of old people to psychiatric hospitals from 1970 onwards. This change is in no way related to the pattern of need of the community and presumably reflects the long-cherished and probably misconceived desire of central government to close psychiatric hospitals and the equally long-cherished desire of some consultant psychiatrists to avoid providing care (other than domiciliary visits) for the elderly. A particular significance of the phenomenon is the resulting influx of demented old people into residential homes where they may cause disruption and considerable administrative uncertainty about how best to accommodate them.[1]

In non-psychiatric hospitals the rising demand among the elderly has been largely contained by a progressive reduction in mean length of stay. Figure 11.1, based on Hospital In-Patient Enquiry (HIPE) data for England and Wales, shows that from 1962 until the early 1970s the elderly showed the same proportional decline in mean length of stay as other age groups. These trends enabled increased demand by the elderly to be accommodated, partly directly and partly by transference of use of hospital resources from younger age groups to the elderly. In 1966 44.9 per cent of all bed days were used by persons aged 65 and over, but by 1975 this proportion had risen to 51.6 per cent. Inspection of Figure 11.1 suggests that the trend of diminishing mean length of stay may now be levelling out and there are probably several factors contributing to this. For patients aged over 65 the changing age structure of the population with a disproportionate increase in very old people is having an effect. Duration of stay among patients aged 75 and over is almost twice that among patients aged 65 to 74 and the ratio of number of patients in these two age groups is increasing, having risen from 0.81 in 1970 to 0.90 in 1975. Second, there are for all age groups some clinical conditions for which the limit of feasibility or safety in

**Figure 11.1: Hospital In-Patient Enquiry (HIPE) Data for England and Wales: Mean Duration of Stay (All Departments) by Age Group, 1962-75 (note logarithmic ordinate)**

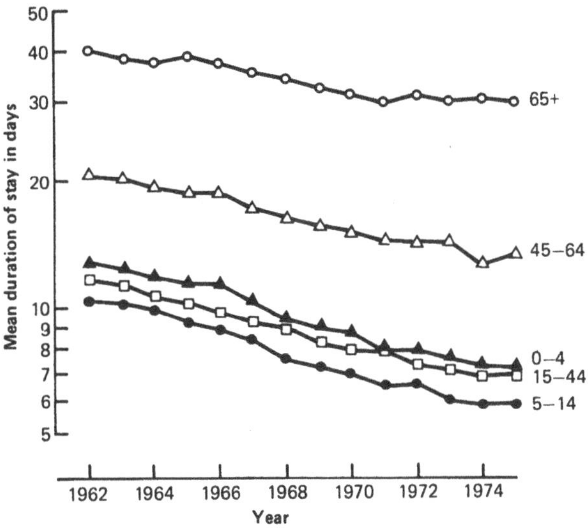


reduction of length of stay may have been reached. The massive reduction in length of hospital stay for treatment of acute myocardial infarction over the last decade is unlikely to continue and the trend towards early discharge of patients following elective surgery is opposed by increased complication rates and the unwillingness of primary care teams to take responsibility for the treatment and supervision devolved from hospital. A third factor, one must regretfully suspect, is a loss of morale among hospital staff who see little incentive to make the efforts required to improve patient throughput. Contributing to this loss of morale are the widening disparities in the distribution of work-load and responsibility compared with that of salaries in the different branches of the Health Service and a growing sense of alienation from the Byzantine complexities of Health Service policies and administration.

If the levelling out of mean duration of stay is a true and permanent feature, it presages a crisis in the hospital service which could only be eased by an expansion in resources or by the introduction of new approaches to improving efficiency or reducing demand. Although the capacity of the National Health Service for 'muddling through' is internationally recognised,[11] the challenges of the next decade will require some more sharply focused policy.

**Table 11.1: Data from the Hospital In-Patient Enquiry for 1966 and 1975 for persons aged 65 and over (England and Wales)**

| All Specialities | 1966 | 1975 | Percentage Change |
|---|---|---|---|
| Discharge rate/$10^4$ | 1,388 | 1,634 | +18 |
| Mean duration of stay (days) | 38 | 31 | -19 |
| Beds per day | 85,510 | 95,940 | +12 |
| Beds per day per $10^6$ | 14,441 | 13,768 | - 4 |
| All Medical Specialities | | | |
| Discharge rate/$10^4$ | 732 | 794 | + 9 |
| Mean duration of stay | 58 | 45 | -21 |
| Beds per day | 74,146 | 68,695 | - 7 |
| Beds per day per $10^6$ | 12,521 | 9,858 | -21 |
| General Surgery with Urology | | | |
| Discharge rate/$10^4$ | 352 | 402 | +14 |
| Mean duration of stay | 19 | 15 | -12 |
| Beds per day | 9,999 | 11,220 | +12 |
| Beds per day per $10^6$ | 1,689 | 1,610 | - 5 |
| Traumatic and Orthopaedic Surgery | | | |
| Discharge rate/$10^4$ | 102 | 143 | +40 |
| Mean duration of stay | 31 | 27 | -14 |
| Beds per day | 5,196 | 7,386 | +42 |
| Beds per day per $10^6$ | 878 | 1,060 | +21 |
| Ophthalmology | | | |
| Discharge rate/$10^4$ | 63 | 62 | - 1 |
| Mean duration of stay | 15 | 11 | -26 |
| Beds per day | 1,476 | 1,273 | -14 |
| Beds per day per $10^6$ | 249 | 183 | -27 |

Concealed in the overall data of Figure 11.1 are some intriguing differences between specialities. Table 11.1 shows the percentage changes in discharge rates, mean duration of stay and average beds occupied daily per million population for persons aged 65 and over in different hospital specialities from 1966 to 1975. The striking anomaly in the table is the performance of traumatic and orthopaedic surgery which has shown an increase in discharge rates which is four times the mean for all specialities but a reduction in mean length of stay which is only two-thirds of that shown by all specialities combined. The number of orthopaedic beds occupied daily has in consequence risen by a fifth compared with a 4 per cent reduction in all specialities combined. This increase in occupied beds has been achieved partly by the practice of boarding out patients to beds of other specialities, but despite this transfer of resources waiting lists for orthopaedic departments have grown to levels causing national concern. Part of the problem undoubtedly arises through the increased demand for elective joint surgery following the technical improvements in this field. Also contributing is an increase in admissions for trauma among the elderly. Despite suggestions to the contrary,[12] there is little evidence for an increase in the age-specific incidence rate of fractures of the proximal femur[13] and one must suspect that the changing age structure of the elderly population and the loss of family nursing care for minor injuries are mainly responsible.

It has been suggested that co-operation between orthopaedic and geriatric departments might improve the functioning of an orthopaedic service,[14] but it is not clear to what extent this improvement is achieved merely by effective transfer of geriatric resources to the use of orthopaedic patients as distinct from a true reduction in overall length of stay. If the former, there is little scope for immediate improvement on a national scale, since geriatric units run at an average occupancy of 92 per cent, which is probably the upper limit of practicability. If, on the other hand, it is the availability of geriatric expertise which is relevant, other possibilities merit consideration, including the introduction of geriatricians as equal partners in orthopaedic teams or the inclusion of geriatric medicine in the postgraduate training of orthopaedic surgeons and nurses.

Clearly the relevance of these alternatives to the plight of orthopaedic units can only be determined by more detailed comparison of services with different working relationships with geriatric services, but it is of interest that some analogous speculations arise in the equally ambiguous border zone between geriatric and general medicine. As Table 11.1 shows, over the decade from 1966 to 1975 these specialities achieved a 22 per cent reduction in the number of beds occupied daily per million population of persons aged 65 and over despite a 7 per cent increase in overall discharge rate. This increase in discharge rate is greater than would have been expected on the basis of the change in age structure of the population between 1966 and 1975, but is considerably less than that observed for all specialities combined. This may be an indication of the extent to which intensifying activity in geriatric day hospitals out-patients, together with the expansion in domiciliary services, has retarded the increase in demand for hospital medical beds for the elderly.

Within the medical specialities the contribution of geriatric units to the care of the elderly is increasing. In 1971, 33 per cent of all medical discharges of elderly people were from geriatric or chronic sick units and these units provided 77 per cent of all medical bed-days used by the elderly. By 1975, although the proportion of medical bed-days provided by geriatric units (chronic sick units no longer being separately categorised) had shown negligible change at 78 per cent, the proportion of all medical discharges that were from geriatric units had risen to 38 per cent. At ages 65 to 74 discharge rates from geriatric units increased by 35 per cent between 1971 and 1975 compared with 7 per cent for other medical specialities. At ages 75 and over the differences are even more dramatic, in that geriatric discharge rates increased by 48 per cent while rates in other medical specialities showed no change. In this age group in 1975 discharge rates from geriatric units were 41 per cent higher than the rates from all other medical specialities combined. It is unfortunately not possible to deduce how much of this increase in discharge rates from geriatric units reflects changes in readmission rates or in transfers between hospitals. The figures do, however, suggest that strident and sometimes uncritical protests about 'bed-blocking' elderly people in non-geriatric units[15] do not arise because of lack of effort by geriatric services.

There seems little reason to doubt that a significant part of the increasing discharge rates from geriatric units is due to a growth in the role of geriatric medicine as a service of primary referral and this is to be seen in the context of the historical development of the speciality. Although we pay just homage to prophets and pioneers such as Marjory Warren, who recognised and responded to the plight of elderly patients before the Second World War, the effective origin of geriatric medicine was in the early years of the National Health Service. An unpropitious origin it was too, owing more to over-recruitment into the training grades of hospital medicine and to the politics of private practice than to any concern by the professional establishment about the welfare of elderly patients. Originally, geriatricians were intended to concern themselves primarily if not exclusively with the supervision of long-stay hospital care for patients transferred from other consultants' services. It quickly became apparent that a significant proportion of patients in long-term hospital care or referred for it were capable of living outside hospital if appropriately managed and so geriatric services developed a rehabilitative function. More recently it has been recognised that consultants in the geriatric service have a role in the hospital care of the acutely ill elderly patient, a role which was accepted implicitly in the report of the Royal College of Physicians Working Party on Medical Care of the Elderly.[16]

For many years geriatric services have in most districts worked in informal partnership with other specialities with no rigorous definition of the separate responsibilities of geriatric or general medical units towards old people referred for admission. In the last five years government policy decisions to give priority in the allocation of resources to the 'geriatric' in preference to the 'acute' sector of non-psychiatric hospital care have precipitated concern that the relationship between geriatric medicine and other medical specialities should be more clearly defined. This is also necessary from the general practitioner's point of view so that he can know which service will accept responsibility for providing care for an individual elderly patient. Too often, it seems, an elderly patient can be regarded as the other services' responsibility by both geriatric and general medical units.

Historically, the specific responsibilities of the geriatric service are contained within the needs of the population aged 65 and over, which forms the planning base for allocation of geriatric resources. Clearly, however, other specialist medical and surgical services must contribute to care of the older population and the overall pattern of provision of hospital care should be appropriate for the needs of the population served. Some of the salient features of illness in the elderly which need to be reflected in available facilities are:

A. multiple pathology;
B. non-specific or atypical presentation of disease;
C. rapid deterioration of illness if untreated;
D. high incidence of secondary complications;
E. prolonged recovery phase;
F. importance of ecological factors – housing, income, social support etc.

(C–F) All features reflecting impairment of homeostatic mechanisms.

To these features characteristic of the patient we may add some practical considerations, for example:

G. the administrative complexity of providing adequate community support;
H. the economic restraints which necessitate optimal deployment of restricted resources;

and finally some longer-term concerns such as:

I. recruitment and training of personnel;
J. fostering appropriate research and development.

Because (A) assessment and supervision by doctors and nurses with appropriately generalist expertise is essential, and because of (A) and (B) the initial assessment of an elderly patient requires full access to modern diagnostic facilities. Because of (C) access to such facilities needs to be immediate and investigation completed as rapidly as possible. These conditions put significant constraints on management of elderly patients in general practice and from a hospital point of view they require that an ill old person needs to be admitted to a unit with district general hospital (DGH) facilities rather than to a unit in a peripheral hospital. The implication is also that the decision that a particular elderly patient would not benefit from DGH investigation and can therefore be admitted directly to a peripheral hospital unit for custodial care can rarely be made safely in the patient's home by even the most experienced physician. Nor, *a fortiori*, can it safely be made by a pre-registration house officer in telephone conversation with a doctors' deputising service.

Although the availability of DGH beds in the medical care of elderly patients is urged in the official recommendation that at least half of the beds of the geriatric service should be on the DGH site,[17] many administrators and doctors seem to assume that this recommendation has more to do with improving the status and morale of geriatricians than with practical service needs. Is there any evidence that DGH medical beds are as significant to the proper functioning of hospital services for the elderly as the theoretical considerations presented above would suggest?

In principle a nation-wide survey of the functioning of services with different patterns of resource provision might provide the necessary information. Recent studies in Newcastle have shown considerable practical difficulties in this approach, including the absence of operational criteria for evaluating the quality of the service, the problem of cross-boundary flows for elderly patients in different specialities and a wide variation in admission rates which raises the possibility that one might not be comparing like with like in terms of need and demand. However, three geriatric services which claim to be successful in providing immediate admission without waiting list and generating minimal numbers of long-stay hospital patients have been described in sufficient detail to permit analysis of the resources used. These services are at Sunderland,[18] Oldham[19] and Hull.[20] Sunderland and Oldham geriatric services provide comprehensive medical care for all persons aged 65 and over but with different management policies. At Oldham initial assessment of patients referred for hospital opinion is based primarily on home visiting, while at Sunderland assessment is made by immediate out-patient attendance. Hull provides a comprehensive medical service for patients aged 75 and over and for younger patients who would benefit from geriatric facilities, but the majority of medical care for persons aged 65 to 74 is provided in other medical departments. In interpreting the success of these services it is necessary to relate their resources to national figures. This is rendered difficult by the unavailability of some data on a national basis and also by the different dates of the three reports, since recent years have seen important trends in the hospital care of elderly patients. We have therefore had to draw on a variety of sources to provide appropriate reference figures, including Hospital In-Patient Enquiry, SH3 returns[21,22] and a postal survey of consultant geriatricians in England and Wales.[23]

Table 11.2 shows the total number of geriatric beds per 1,000 persons aged 65 and over in the population served. Provision at two of the centres is higher than the national average. The provision in Hull of 8.1 beds per 1,000 was based on 1971 populations and may be an overestimate by about 7 per cent.[24] More striking in Table 11.2 is the comparison of geriatric beds associated with general hospital facilities with

**Table 11.2: Comparative Statistics for Three Successful Geriatric Services**

| | Hull 1974 | Oldham 1972 | Sunderland 1971 | Reference Figures[a] |
|---|---|---|---|---|
| A Geriatric beds per 1,000 elderly[a] | 8.1 | 9.1 | 9.0 | 8.6 |
| B Geriatric beds with general hospital facilities | 5.7 | 8.5 | 8.5 | 2.8 |
| C Percentage of geriatric beds with general hospital facilities | 70 | 93 | 92 | 33 |
| D Geriatric plus medical beds available to the elderly per 1,000 | 11.1 | 9.6 | 10.0 | 11.2 |
| E Total medical beds with general hospital facilities available for the elderly per 1,000 (B + (D – A)) | 8.7 | 9.0 | 9.5 | 5.4 |
| F Total medical specialities admission rate per 1,000 elderly per year | 123 | 60 | 82 | 74 (1971)<br>78 (1974) |

Note: a. See text.

which all three centres are generously provided. The classification of beds as having general hospital facilities is necessarily somewhat arbitrary: we have taken as a minimal definition the presence of junior medical staff, the availability of a full range of laboratory investigation with return of results on the same day and radiographic facilities including barium studies available on site daily. Owing to progressive upgrading of facilities in Hull since 1970, 70 per cent is a minimal estimate of the proportion of geriatric beds there which have general hospital facilities. No official national figures were available using comparable definitions, but for comparison we present the overall figures revealed by replies from 108 districts of England in response to a postal questionnaire of consultant geriatricians.[23] The figures obtained from this survey were higher than those found in a more detailed study of geriatric services in the northern region.[25]

The 'subsidy' to geriatric services from beds available to the elderly in other medical units is obviously an important factor to be considered. We have calculated this for Sunderland from bed occupancy figures based on average beds occupied daily, adding an increment corresponding to a bed occupancy rate of 76 per cent to approximate the national occupancy for non-geriatric medical beds in 1971. For Hull and Oldham we have taken the published numbers of admissions to non-geriatric medical units and have applied an estimated mean length of stay of 15 days. The mean length of stay in patients aged 65 to 74 in general medical units was 18 days during 1972-4. Our estimated value of 15 has been based on the assumption that longer-stay patients will have been filtered off to the geriatric services in Hull and Oldham, but that some of the patients in the non-geriatric units will be of an older age group or allocated to chest medicine, both categories being associated with longer mean length of stay. Again an increment has been added to the calculated daily beds occupied to allow for an estimated bed occupancy of 76 per cent, thus converting beds occupied by persons aged over 65 to beds available to this age group. Obviously 'availability' in this context is a statistical concept which may or may not correspond to the ease with which elderly patients obtain access to these beds. Medical bed occupancy in Hull is, in fact, somewhat lower than 76 per cent.[24] In deriving national figures for comparison we have used 1974 HIPE estimates of number of admissions and mean duration of stay with the additional assumption of 92 per cent average occupancy in geriatric departments and 76 per cent in other units. By adding the geriatric beds with general hospital facilities to the non-geriatric medical beds available to the elderly we have estimated the total number of medical beds with DGH facilities available to the elderly. This demonstrates that the average availability of such beds in the three centres is higher than the national average.

Admission rates to all medical specialities (including geriatric medicine) are also presented in Table 11.2 The admission rate at Hull is higher than the national average, but Oldham apparently achieves its successful medical services for the elderly at much lower admission rates. This may reflect the policy at Oldham that referrals are assessed at home before admission is decided upon. There may be important social and economic implications in the resulting differences in admission rate if, as seems likely, these reflect policy rather than morbidity or demand.

The function of hospital medical services for the elderly may depend heavily on psychiatric and social services. Part III accommodation at Hull was provided at 22 places per 1,000 elderly and Oldham at 20 per 1,000, both being relatively high figures for the year reported. Part III accommodation for Sunderland in 1971 was about 18 beds per 1,000. The psychiatric admission rate for persons aged 65 and over in Hull was reported as 5.7 per 1,000 per year, which may be compared with the national figure of 3.2 per 1,000 per year.[26] Corresponding data for Oldham and Sunderland are not published.

These data are clearly incomplete and reflect the inadequacy of information available on the performance of successful geriatric services. Important elements in running a hospital service are the degree of co-operation with social services and with psychiatric departments. In particular, a geriatric service whose social service colleagues will accept incontinent or confused patients to Part III homes will have fewer long-stay patients in hospital beds. No information on social services policy in this important regard is provided in the three reports analysed. None-the less, although it has been claimed that the ability to run a successful geriatric service depends primarily on attitudes and policies,[27] our findings are compatible with the view that the success of services at Hull, Oldham and Sunderland is made possible by the generous provision of resources, particularly DGH beds, in which the three districts are similar rather than to management policies in which they differ. This is not, however, to suggest that resources will run themselves and the personal achievements of the geriatric teams in these three districts are outstanding.

If it is a correct postulate that it is a high number of DGH beds available to the elderly which enables a successful medical service to be provided, the next obvious question is whether it is also necessary for a large proportion of these beds to be in the 'geriatric' rather than the 'general medical' allocation. There is evidence that specialist geriatricians can contribute to the management of elderly patients in non-geriatric wards. Burley *et al.*[28] demonstrated that the formal attachment of a consultant geriatrician to medical units reduces the length of stay of elderly patients independently of transfer to geriatric beds and similar observations have been made in Newcastle. Our personal interpretation of this finding is that it does not arise from better treatment of patients in a strictly medical sense, but from more efficient management arising from experience of, and involvement in, the full range of medical services available to the elderly. The efficiency of management in this sense involves both medical and nursing staff. This interpretation is supported by some studies of 'bed-blocking', which indicate that some elderly patients may be mismanaged in non-geriatric units through unawareness of the services available and of the need to form a realistic and forward-looking plan of management for elderly patients.[29] In other words, not only do the elderly need access to DGH medical beds, if the management of their illnesses is to be maximally efficient they need also to encounter appropriate medical and nursing expertise which may not always be available in non-geriatric units as currently organised. The desirable combination of resources and expertise can, however, be provided in more than one way and we return to this later.

The aspects of care discussed in the last paragraph clearly relate to items (F) and (G) in the features of illness in the elderly which we listed earlier – the importance of ecological factors and the administrative complexity of community care. There are also implications for item (H) – the need to minimise cost. Also relevant to the problem of costs is the prolonged recovery phase of illness in the elderly (item E). DGH beds are expensive and we need to know what proportion of medical beds for the elderly can and should be provided in cheaper accommodation. An important factor is the observation that after a prolonged stay, visiting of elderly patients in hospital falls off as a function of travelling distance[30] so that for longer-term rehabilitation and for permanent hospital care beds should be available close to the communities from which the patients have been admitted. Whether this necessitates the provision of beds in community hospitals clearly depends on the geography and transport facilities of particular districts. Table 11.2 suggests that for urban services perhaps only 2 beds per 1,000 should normally be provided in peripheral hospitals compared with the 5.0 permitted by DHSS plans and the present national average of 5.8.

The existence of beds outside the DGH site raises practical problems in their supervision. On medical grounds it is possible to argue that services for patients who cannot be discharged directly from admission unit beds back into the community but need to go for rehabilitation to another hospital would be better if the doctors who provided the acute care were also responsible for the subsequent care. It is only by providing continuity of responsibility in this way that the pattern of care in the acute units can be integrated with that in the longer-stay areas. This integration is necessary to ensure that orientation and methods of treatment are similar throughout the service and that the attitudes of patients and relatives are managed consistently. Integration is also necessary for doctors and nurses to be appropriately appraised of the medium- and long-term outcome of their management. It benefits neither patients nor professions for doctors and nurses to lose sight of their mistakes and failures. This concept of continued responsibility forms, with adequate resources and appropriate expertise, the third essential factor in care for the elderly. Governmental recognition for this emerges in the transmutation of the 'physician with a special interest in geriatric medicine' of the Royal College of Physicians Working Party on Medical Care of the Elderly[16] into the 'physician with a special responsibility for the aged' of a recent DHSS letter to Regional Medical Officers.[31]

In the growing financial crisis in the National Health Service the costs of any increase in hospital bed numbers will need to be kept to a minimum. This inevitably suggests that for the foreseeable future expansion will only take place in 'community hospitals' or other peripheral units. If our reasoning about the importance of DGH beds in the care of the elderly is correct, a policy which permits the expansion of geriatric units only outside DGH sites will not solve the problems of the hospital service. Could it be that the best of some specialities other than geriatric medicine might be more rationally placed in peripheral units?

With regard to the organisation of hospital medical care for the elderly, two basic models have recently emerged. The first is the separatist model taking a defined age as separating the responsibilities of geriatric and general medical services, a model which if associated with appropriate allocation of resources can be highly successful as demonstrated at Hull, Oldham and Sunderland. The second model, which we may call the integrationist approach, is to accept that at least to the end of the century the elderly will be numerically the most important group of patients requiring hospital medical care and that the organisation of general medical units should be adapted accordingly. This will require appropriate training for medical and nursing staff on these units and also that if there are consultants with special responsibility for the elderly they should have their admission beds on the units and be involved in training of unit staff and determining unit policy and organisation. The same consultant should also be responsible for the rehabilitation, long-stay and day hospital facilities available to the units. This approach has been adopted as policy in one or two areas[32] and is facilitated by some of the provisions of the Royal College of Physicians Working Party on Medical Care of the Elderly[16] and some recent DHSS policy,[31] but is not yet of demonstrated efficacy. Among the suggested advantages of the arrangement are an increased efficiency in the use of resources compared with running two parallel age-defined medical services. A further advantage is that it provides postgraduate experience in the case of the elderly under specialist supervision for junior doctors and nurses who may go on to careers which require considerable expertise in the management of elderly patients, but for which no provision is made in postgraduate training for the acquisition of relevant skills. This may have particular relevance for specialities such as orthopaedic surgery whose present plight in attempting to provide care for the elderly was outlined earlier. There is no reason why this advantage could not be embodied in the age-defined geriatric units if rotation of *all* junior staff between non-geriatric and geriatric units were insisted upon. One of the suggested disadvantages of the integrationist approach is that because of traditional professional attitudes the role of the specialist geriatrician could be less than appropriate and that continuity of care would be less than is possible in age-defined units. There is also the anxiety that unless an adequate training in geriatric medicine is insisted upon, consultants appointed to integrationist posts could be seduced by the attractions of the acute aspect of their work and neglect their wider responsibilities to the community.

It could be argued that the logical conclusion of the integrationist approach would be the disappearance of geriatric medicine as a speciality by its absorption into general medicine, an idea which clearly appeals to some.[33] If this occurred, one might reasonably question, in view of present demographic trends, whether it was geriatric or general medicine that had been abolished. Is there indeed a future for general medicine that is not geriatric?

In the longer term recruitment of doctors into hospital care of the elderly is a crucial problem. Over the last decade two-thirds of consultant appointments in geriatric medicine in England and Wales have been of foreign graduates, a proportion much higher than in other major specialities. It is doubtful if the speciality could have survived in its present form and with its present deficiencies without this influx of foreign graduates. Personal experience in undergraduate and post-graduate medical education suggests strongly that the unattractiveness of the speciality is dominantly due to the poor working conditions and inadequate resources provided for most geriatric services. There is also the problem of an excessive work-load. At present consultants in general medicine have an average of around 30 beds under their care. For consultants in geriatric medicine the number is about 180 and the additional commitments of out-patients, day hospitals, community and management work are greater than in most other medical specialities. The low status of the speciality in the profession, which is sometimes suspected as contributing to poor recruitment, is inextricably associated with resource allocation, although an associated factor is the image of the speciality as being concerned only with patients that other specialities have rejected and the isolation of junior medical staff in units away from the DGH and its educational opportunities. Although professonal status, pleasant environment and money contribute to the motivation of doctors in choosing a career, an important aspect of the motivation of hospital doctors is craftsmanship, the reward of providing a good and progressive service to patients individually and collectively. For only a minority of geriatric posts in the United Kingdom are resources sufficient to realise this objective.

The latter part of this essay has been concerned with the future development of non-psychiatric hospital care for the elderly. One may speculate that if economic expansion in the United Kingdom had continued unabated, the contribution of geriatric units to the acute medical care of the elderly would have quietly continued to increase without too much introspection. We have somewhat cynically suggested that it is only the threat of specific allocation of resources away from the more traditional specialities that has precipitated so much recent interest among non-geriatricians in the future of geriatric medicine. The debate is unnecessarily acrimonious and sterile because issues are seen too much in terms of the conflict between professional groups separated by attitudes adopted 25 years ago. These attitudes are no longer appropriate, but continue because both government and professions traditionally think in terms of structure rather than function in their contributions to the organisation of health care. One possible beneficial outcome of our financial difficulties may be the recognition of the principles underlying good-quality care of the elderly and the realisation that these principles can be implemented within a range of different administrative arrangements. The evidence that we have reviewed in this essay shows that the problems of the hospital service in providing care for the elderly can be solved within finite resources. The fear that care of the elderly is a bottomless hole into which any amount of resources could sink without significant effect is unjustified. Unjustified too, as we have pointed out elsewhere,[34] is the idea that providing care for the elderly has made matters worse by reducing mortality rates. The problem will not go away and it can be solved – but only if politicians and public decide it is worth solving.

## References

1. Evans, J. Grimley (1976) 'Issues in Institutional Care in the United Kingdom' in A.N. Exton-Smith and J. Grimley Evans (eds.), *Care of the Elderly. Meeting the Challenge of Dependency*, Academic Press, London, pp. 128-46
2. Department of Health and Social Security (1975) *The Census of Residential Accommodation: 1970. I. Residential Accommodation for the Elderly and for the Younger Physically Handicapped* HMSO, London
3. Wilkin, D., Mashiah, T. and Jolley, D.J. (1978) 'Changes in Behavioural Characteristics of Elderly Populations of Local Authority Homes and Long-stay Hospital Wards 1976-77', *British Medical Journal, 2*, 1274-6
4. Townsend, P. (1962) *The Last Refuge*, Routledge and Kegan Paul, London
5. Thatcher, A.R. (1973) 'Variation of Activity Rates and Earnings with Increasing Age', *Proceedings of the Royal Society of Medicine, 66*, 811-12
6. Government Statistical Service (1976) *Social Trends No. 7*, HMSO London
7. Leader (1979) 'Planning for the Old and Very Old', *British Medical Journal, 2*, 952
8. Robertson, C., Gilmore, A., and Caird, F.I. (1975) 'Demography of Families of the Elderly in Glasgow', *Health Bulletin, 33*, 1-6
9. Brocklehurst, J.C., Carty, M.H., Leeming, J.T., and Robinson, J.M. (1978) 'Medical Screening of Old People Accepted for Residential Care', *Lancet, 2*, 141-3
10. Shulman, K., and Arie, T.H.D. (1978) 'Fall in Admission Rate of Old People to Psychiatric Units', *British Medical Journal, 1*, 156-8
11. Maddox, G.L. (1971) 'Muddling Through: Planning for Health Care in England', *Medical Care, 9*, 439-48
12. Burton, J.L. Ensell, F.J., Leach , J.F., and Hall, K.A. (1975) 'Atmospheric Ozone and Femoral Fractures', *Lancet, 1*, 795-6
13. Evans, J. Grimley, Prudham, D., and Wandless, I. (1979) 'A Prospective Study of Fractured Proximal Femur: Incidence and Outcome', *Public Health, 93*, 235-41
14. Irvine, R.E., and Strouthidis, T.M. (1977) 'The Geriatric Orthopaedic Unit' in M. Devas (ed.), *Geriatric Orthopaedics*, Academic Press, London, pp. 185-94
15. McArdle, C., Wylie, J.C. and Alexander, W.D. (1975) 'Geriatric Patients in an Acute Medical Ward', *British Medical Journal, 4*, 568-9
16. Report of the Working Party of the Royal College of Physicians of London (1977) 'Medical Care of the Elderly', *Lancet, 1*, 1092-5
17. Department of Health and Social Security (1971) *Hospital Services for the*

*Elderly*, DS 329/71

18. Gedling, P., and Newell, D.J. (1972) 'Hospital Beds for the Elderly', in G. McLachlan (ed.), *Problems and Progress in Medical Care. Seventh Series*, Oxford University Press, Oxford
19. O'Brien, T.D., Joshi, D.M., and Warren, E.W. (1973) 'No Apology for Geriatrics', *British Medical Journal, 4*, 277-80
20. Bagnall, W.E., Datta, S.R., Knox, J., and Horrocks, P. (1977) 'Geriatric Medicine in Hull: a Comprehensive Service', *British Medical Journal, 2*, 102-4
21. Report on Hospital In-Patient Enquiry *HMSO London*
22. *Department of Health and Social Security Annual Reports*, HMSO London
23. Evans, J. Grimley (1979) (unpublished)
24. Horrocks, P. (1979) personal communication
25. *Northern Region Sub-committee on Geriatric Medicine* (unpublished)
26. Department of Health and Social Security (1977) 'In-patient Statistics from the Mental Health Enquiry for England, 1974', *Statistical and Research Report Series No. 17*, HMSO London
27. Hodkinson, H.M. and Jefferys, P.M. (1972) 'Making Hospital Geriatrics Work', *British Medical Journal, 4*, 536-9
28. Burley, L.E., Currie, C.T., Smith, R.G., and Williamson, J. (1979) 'Contribution from Geriatric Medicine within Acute Medical Wards', *British Medical Journal, 2*, 90-2
29. Rubin, S.G., and Davies, G.M. (1975) 'Bed-blocking by Elderly Patients in General Hospital Wards', *Age and Ageing, 4*, 142-7
30. Cross, K.W., and Turner, R.D. (1974) 'Factors Affecting the Visiting Pattern of Geriatric Patients in a Rural Area', *British Journal of Preventive and Social Medicine, 28*, 133-9
31. Department of Health and Society Security (1979) 'Physicians in Geriatric Medicine and Physicians with a Special Responsibility for the Aged', letter to Regional Medical Officers, B/M169/6D
32. Evans, J. Grimley (1974) 'Geriatrics', *Lancet, 2*, 282-3
33. Leonard, J.C. (1976) 'Can Geriatrics Survive?' *British Medical Journal, 1*, 1335-6
34. Evans, J. Grimley (1978) 'Demography and Resources', *Medicine, 3*, 12-14

# 12 SCREENING, SURVEILLANCE AND CASE-FINDING

J. Williamson

> The reafons why Perfons in this Age fall fo foon into this decrepit ftate, and why the miferies thereof are fo multiplied and magnified upon them, is, becaufe either they call not in foon enough for help, or becaufe thofe that are called in either underftand not, or minde not what they ought to do. An honeft and an able Phyfician, may furely approve himfelf to his ancient Patient (as Ruth's Son was to his Grandmother). A reftorer of life, and nourifher of old age.
>
> John Smith, MD
> *The Pourtract of Old Age*
> Feb. 17. 1676

My interest in preventive aspects of geriatric care, and especially in screening and case-finding, was aroused as soon as I became interested in care of the elderly. The year was 1958, until when I had been a consultant in respiratory diseases with special responsibility for the central chest clinic in Edinburgh. This clinic was situated in the Royal Victoria Dispensary which was the descendant of the pioneering tuberculosis dispensary founded in the city by Sir Robert Philip in 1887. Sir Robert's original conception of tuberculosis control was based upon prevention, early diagnosis and effective treatment, and underlying it all was the realisation of the fundamental importance of social factors both in prevention and in determining response to treatment. For the recovering patient, rehabilitation and reintroduction to normal social life were essential and these aspects were given priority and introduced at an early stage.

As a student and young doctor I had been only too well aware of the despair which was associated with a diagnosis of 'TB', and it was a remarkable privilege to have worked in a busy chest clinic during the fifties when this 'Captain of the Men of Death' was brought to his knees as the epidemic came under effective control.

It was with optimism, therefore, that I approached my new career in geriatric medicine, filled with enthusiasm (and perhaps arrogance) and in the belief that having defeated one apparently insuperable enemy, old age and its ill effects could likewise be coped with! Now, several decades later, and hopefully much wiser, I still feel that there is much to be optimistic about in the care of the elderly and I am more than ever convinced that the greatest opportunities lie in the fields of prevention and earlier case-finding.

It did not take long to discover that there was to be no magical chemotherapy for cure as in the case of tuberculosis, as many of the pathological conditions encountered were degenerative in nature and thus not amenable to cure. At the same time, however, I realised that even if the underlying conditions could not be influenced, the resulting disabilities very often could, by rational therapies and by rehabilitation. In a large majority some function could be restored and in practically all the progress could be slowed. This required a major adjustment in approach and one learned to think much more in terms of function (lost, preserved and regained) rather than in the classical fashion of pathology first and last. In addition, it was very easy to see the importance of social factors such as loneliness and isolation in leading to low morale and apathy and thus in increasing dependency. The value of adequate social services was thus readily appreciated.

In all these matters, the need for early diagnosis and early detection of loss of physical, mental or social function seemed of paramount importance, and it was seen as an affront to have an old lady with disabling arthritis referred to the geriatric service only after she had become immobilised with limb weakness and joint contractures and when her caring daughter had become exhausted with the burden of looking after her. Likewise it seemed irrational and wasteful to have a stroke victim referred 'for addition to your long-term waiting list' perhaps months or even years after the cerebrovascular accident. So often the referring doctor described the exhausted daughter as being 'at the end of her tether' or sometimes even more illogically as 'rejecting' the patient. It soon became clear that, as far as supporting family members were concerned, once they had been taken beyond their limits of tolerance, rejection would occur and once this had been allowed to happen, the rupture was generally irreversible. Thus the daughter who had been reduced to an exhausted, irritable and bad-tempered wreck would never allow herself to be exposed to this hazard again. This seemed to me to have the greatest significance for the happiness and well-being of old people, for their families and, in addition, for the hard-pressed and invariably limited services which were struggling to cope with the complex problems of an ageing population in modern society.

During 1962-3 we conducted a research study upon 200 persons aged 65 and over, selected at random from three local practices. The objective was to determine the amount and nature of disability in these subjects and to find out how much of this was known to the relevant general practitioner. The outcome was that subjects tended to have multiple disabilities (about three per person) and for every one that was known to the GP there was another which was not.[1] More detailed analysis of the findings showed that there was a pattern about the 'iceberg' of unknown disabilities. Figure 12.1 shows the proportion of known and unknown disabilities which related to the cardiovascular system, the respiratory system and the central nervous system.

**Figure 12.1: Unknown Disabilities in Older Persons: Disabilities in which Most of the Iceberg is above Water (practitioner's awareness is relatively high)**

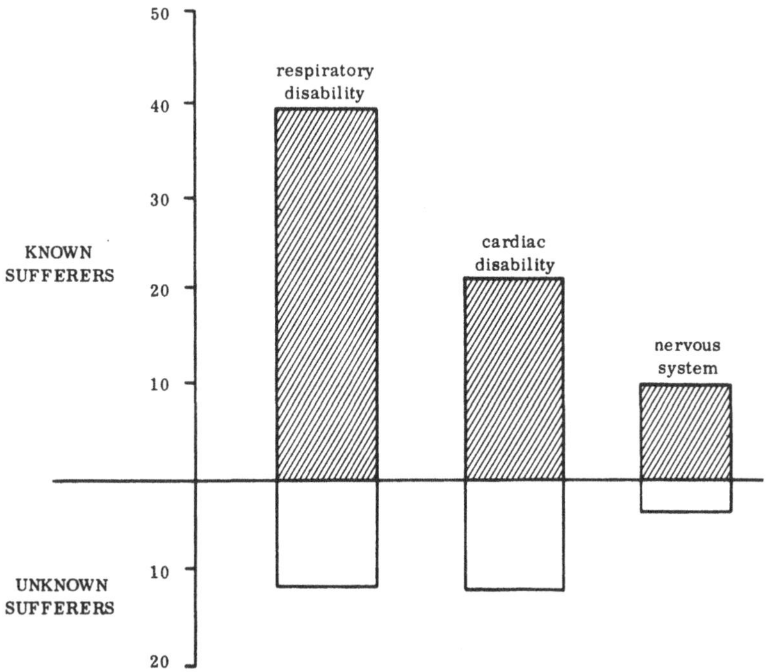


It will be seen that these disabilities tended to be well known to general practitioners and it seemed that old people therefore realised that cough, expectoration, breathlessness or loss of power in a limb were symptoms which ought to be referred to a doctor. Perhaps this was partly because doctors tended to be more interested and helpful about such complaints?

In marked contrast, however, were the findings in relation to other important disabilities, especially those associated with disease of joints, feet, urinary tract and with mental illness (especially dementia). Figure 12.2 shows the high proportion of unknown disabilities in these systems.

**Figure 12.2: Unknown Disabilities in Older Persons: Disabilities in which Most of the Iceberg is Submerged (practitioner's awareness is low)**

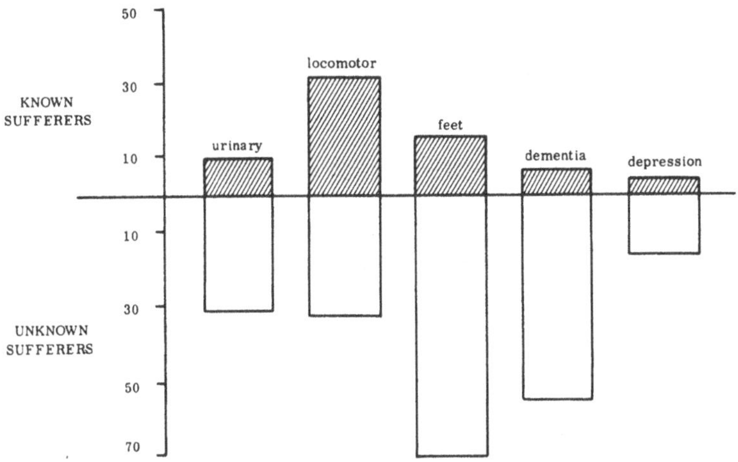


It is interesting to note that these largely unknown disabilities are of great importance for the affected individual and possess special implications. Thus locomotor disabilities are painful and progressive and they lead to restriction of mobility. Hence they may readily lead to impoverishment of social activity, difficulty in shopping and hence carry the danger of producing social isolation and loneliness and eventually apathy and risk of malnutrition. The onset of bladder dysfunction, in males post-micturition dribbling and in females stress incontinence and precipitancy, lead to considerable distress and embarrassment. The old lady who dare not allow herself to be more than a few yards from a toilet, or the old man whose underclothes are frequently wet with urine, may often react by limitation of social life and consequent dangers of isolation and low morale. Pehaps the greatest risk, however, is for the elderly dementing patient whose condition goes undetected until a late stage. It is sometimes argued that this makes little practical difference since the great majority of patients suffering from dementia are affected by Alzheimer primary neuronal degeneration or arteriopathic, multi-infarct disease and there is no cure or effective therapy for either type. So what difference does it make whether their condition is known or not?

To pose such a question reveals profound ignorance of the condition and its consequences. Thus, the old lady who is quietly dementing, who retains her equable temperament and is safely supported by a 'normal' family structure will present few problems, since her daughters will instinctively support her while encouraging her to pursue her remaining useful roles – washing dishes, light housework, preparing vegetables, etc. These activities not only afford the patient substantial satisfaction but also secure healthy tiredness and hence peaceful nights. Indeed the physical energy thus usefully employed may be of practical value to the family. If, however, the lady is living alone and is unsupported she is at great risk because of her reduced social competence, her inability to make rational judgements and her lack of insight into the nature and seriousness of her predicament. She is thus liable to secondary consequences of malnutrition and self-neglect and if there is a behaviour disturbance such as restlessness, wandering, 'turning night into day', repetitive questioning and searching and bouts of aggression, even the most caring relatives and sympathetic neighbours will soon reach 'the end of their tether'. It becomes, therefore, a matter of the greatest urgency that such patients should be identified at the earliest stage so that, after full assessment, suitable measures may be instituted to ensure that the patient is adequately supported and necessary services supplied. Help is also essential for relatives and others involved with the patient and this may vary from sympathetic listening and counselling to repeated respite admission and regular day care.

## The Reasons for Non-reporting of Disability in Old Age

Why is it that many old people seem to behave in this rather irrational and obstinate fashion and fail to report significant disabilities to their doctors or to other primary care workers? The reasons are complex and multiple. There is the fatalism of old people which leads them to say, 'It's all due to my age' or 'My doctor is a busy person and he must have more important patients to worry about' or 'There's not much can be done at my age anyway.' These common statements help to explain why many old people with bladder problems fail to consult their doctors – 'I thought that all old men got this sort of trouble.' Similarly, old people with painful foot conditions clain that they thought little could be done since all old people suffered this way sooner or later, often despite the fact that simple chiropody would effect immediate substantial relief. Then there is the element of fear of the consequences of diagnosis and it seems likely that some old people are afraid that if they go to a doctor the ensuing diagnosis may lead to hospital admission or admission to residential care. The underlying, often unformulated, fear is of a loss of independence and the danger that others may take over the control of their lives – a control which may be difficult to regain once lost. Perhaps the present generation of old people are significantly influenced in their attitude to seeking medical help by the fact that during their formative early years going to a doctor was often a luxury which they would only have sought for major problems and certainly not for relative trivialities such as stiff joints or 'bladder weakness'. Maybe future generations of old people who have been conditioned to use comprehensive health services will behave differently and some have claimed that this is already occurring in the younger old persons of today.

In addition to these factors, older people have fewer incentives to report illness. Thus the younger man views disability as a threat to his earning capacity and his employability, while the younger woman sees her important roles as mother and family manager threatened. For the old man the pension continues whether he is disabled or not and for the ageing widow there are often no dependants for her to worry about, so these incentives, which may drive younger persons to seek medical help, are inoperative in old age.

## The Rationale of Screening and Surveillance

In the opening paragraph in our paper on 'Unreported Needs'[1] we stated:

> One of the most striking and distressing features of work in a geriatric unit is that patients are so often admitted in a very advanced stage of disease. Many have pressure sores or permanent joint contractures and show signs of prolonged neglect and subnutrition. Yet the family doctor may write 'I saw this patient for the first time yesterday' or 'the last time I saw this old lady was two years ago when her husband died'. Careful history taking will establish that timely medical or social intervention might have prevented much of this disability. Why then was it not forthcoming?

This thought had prompted the study reported in *The Lancet* and it is gratifying to report that there has been a substantial improvement since those dark days of nearly twenty years ago in Edinburgh. No longer is it common to have patients referred in such an advanced stage of disability, nor is it at all common to find limb contractures and gross self-neglect. One can only feel grateful that these improvements have occurred.

A plea was made in the 1964 article that general practitioners should make special efforts to keep in touch with their old patients and that health visitors should 'undertake periodic visiting of old people and carry out screening' and 'ascertain the degree of mobility of the old person and enquire into the cause of any deterioration'.

Since that time much attention has been paid to 'geriatric screening' and many studies have been reported, usually with similar findings of a large iceberg of undeclared disability and morbidity. It has also often been postulated that detection of this 'iceberg' is possible by systematic search and that cure or alleviation will often result.

In the Kilsyth study[2] it was revealed that about one-third of needs detected in the survey were unknown and, although some of these conditions were not severe, many were of a progressive nature and were linked with the liability of loss of mobility, lowered self-esteem and erosion of independence. The earlier Edinburgh study[1] had shown that one-fifth of undetected disabilities were severe and Akhtar and his colleagues[3] emphasised the rapid increase in prevalence of major disability which occurred with age. By age 85, about four out of five persons were thus afflicted. Other surveys have confirmed these general findings, notably those of Thomas (1968),[4] Burns (1969),[5] Currie and colleagues (1974)[6] and Barber and Wallis (1976).[7]

There has therefore developed a considerable body of opinion that 'geriatric screening' is a worthwhile activity and it ought to be encouraged. Unfortunately, however, the situation remains confused, first because there is no agreement as to what 'screening' really means and, second, because no one has yet scientifically evaluated it or even determined who ought to be performing it.

One attempt at evaluation was that of Lowther and his colleagues,[8] in which 300 patients were followed up after being involved in a scheme of health visitor case-finding and attendance at a geriatric consultative clinic. The period of follow-up varied from 18 to 30 months and 29 per cent were then adjudged still to be benefiting from the results of the screening procedure. Williams[9] reviewed 200 patients one year after screening and concluded that only 8 per cent could be said to have received lasting benefit from specific therapy. These studies were uncontrolled and the criteria were subjective, and the best that one can conclude upon the benefits of screening must at present be 'not proven'.

Despite this lack of evidence of benefit, health visitors, general practitioners and other health workers have tended to accept that this activity represents worthwhile use of resources and the cry for more screening facilities is often heard. Thus Age Concern, in its report of 1978,[10] states unequivocally: 'We strongly encourage the development of screening facilities for regular check-ups of elderly people who want this both at hospital and by family practitioners.'

It appears therefore that a stage has been reached at which it is essential to clarify these issues and to determine answers to the following questions:

(1) What do we mean by 'geriatric screening' and what should be the content of screening programmes?
(2) Who should carry it out?
(3) Which elderly persons should be screened?
(4) What is the value to the individual old person of this activity in improved health, well-being and independence?
(5) What is the cost-effectiveness of this procedure and what priority should it be accorded in the provision of health services?

Sadly, it must be admitted that we have either no answer or only partial answers to all these important questions.

## What do we Mean by 'Geriatric Screening' and What should be the Content of Screening Programmes?

It is important here to be clear about terminology since some of the present confusion has been caused by imprecision.

I should like to suggest that instead of using the term 'screening', we ought now to be referring to 'case-finding'. In the document *Prevention and Health*[11] it is stated: 'Screening differs from ordinary clinical practice in that it involves seeking out people with no overt symptoms of disease and asking them to undergo examination and tests to see whether the condition to be identified is present.' It may therefore be seen that measures directed at the detection of unreported illness or established disability are not included within this definition of screening since the latter is concerned only with those 'with no overt symptoms of disease'. It may be argued, of course, that patients' awareness of their disabilities and their willingness to report them is the criterion by which they may be judged 'overt' or not. The argument now becomes rather circular and sterile, but the pragmatist ought to have little difficulty in deciding what is overt and what is not and thus in distinguishing true screening from what ought more correctly to be described as case-finding. Put in another way, screening is a form of secondary prevention, i.e. the search for precursors of disease in those who do not have the symptoms of the disease and who believe themselves to be free from it. Case-finding, on the other hand is a form of tertiary prevention in which established disease and resultant disability are sought in order to achieve earlier diagnosis and thus create better prospects for care (or alleviation) and rehabilitation.

The practical importance of making this distinction is increased if emphasis is placed upon the detection of loss of function rather than the detection of pathological states or their biochemical or laboratory precursors. In geriatric medicine, one of the important principles is to think in terms of function since, in the majority of cases, the underlying pathology is degenerative and therefore not amenable to cure, or even to modification by therapeutic measures. The resulting loss of function, however, is usually capable of being reduced by rehabilitation, and support may readily be provided to compensate for inability to perform some of the essential tasks of daily living. To emphasise, early detection of loss of function has the additional advantage of broadening the search to include not only loss of physical and mental function but also of social function, impairment of which is just as significant in determining whether an old person will cope adequately with life's demands or head for increasing dependency. Viewed in this way, case-finding ought to encompass search for loss of mobility, loss of vision and hearing, loss of postural control, loss of memory and in addition specific enquiry as to which social activities are impaired or reduced.

Screening of the type defined above (search for non-overt) has become very fashionable in some parts of the world, especially North America and France, and the term multiphasic screening has been introduced to describe a range of screening tests applied during one attendance of the subject at the screening centre. Some writers[12] have cast serious doubt upon the value of screening and yet its spread appears to be continuing. It seems that this is an activity which is both popular with sections of the medical profession and with influential groups within the general public. One of the earliest and most publicised exercises in multiphasic screening has been at the Kaiser Permanente Center in Oakland, California. Reports from this centre, however, have failed to show significant differences between screened and control groups in terms of mortality rates up to seven years after screening. The screened group showed significantly lower rates of self-assessed disability and less time off work than controls, and for certain arbitrarily classified conditions, early detection of which might reasonably be expected to reduce mortality (hypertension-related conditions, cancer of large bowel, rectum, breast, cervix, uterus, kidney and prostate), there was a reduced death rate in the screened group ($p < 0.05$).[13] This study has several important defects and its conclusions are open to criticism.

The report from the South East London Screening Group[14] provides a much more scientific evaluation of multiphasic screening and it failed to show significant differences between screened and control groups in hospital admission rates, certified periods of sickness and in mortality in subjects aged 40 to 64 years. Apologists for multiphasic screening have claimed that the reasons for these failures rest not in the screening process itself but in a failure to provide adequate treatment and control of the conditions detected by the tests, i.e. the failure lay with the doctor or doctors to whom the patients with abnormalities were referred and the claim is then that the screening has not therefore been given a 'fair chance' to succeed.

No detailed studies of multiphasic screening have been done in elderly populations, but those who have strayed into the field have been apt to retire in bewilderment at the large range of 'abnormalities' which are uncovered and the problems of knowing what to do about them. Most results in an old population will fall within the 'entirely normal' range and a few will be 'frankly abnormal', but even with some of those it may be difficult to decide what should be done, for example, the finding of a systolic blood pressure of 180 mm Hg in a woman of 80 years, or of a raised cholesterol in a man of 75. A substantial minority may fall into the 'borderline' category, and here special problems and dangers lie. Are these 'borderline abnormals' to be fully investigated, even with invasive techniques? If so, what will this mean in terms of diversion of resources? What are the benefits to the individual old person and what are the dangers, both from the further investigation itself and from the creating of anxiety? There is an ever present danger in old age that inappropriate medical activity may make a 'person' into a 'patient' without any real prospect of benefit.

For these reasons, among others, I would claim that there is at present no justification for multiphasic screening procedures in an elderly population.

Is there a reasonable basis for case-finding or group surveillance in the elderly?[1,15] In these programmes, elderly persons are offered the opportunity to declare symptoms, loss of function and unmet social needs and by simple examination their physical, mental and social disabilities are uncovered.

A good deal of work has now been invested in this kind of surveillance and effectiveness is usually considered under various headings.

## Validity of Screening and Case-finding

Validity means the ability of any procedure to distinguish those who have the condition or disability which is being sought from those who do not. Thus a fully valid procedure would be one which identified all those with the sought defect and excluded all without it. There would thus be zero false positives and zero false negatives. The term sensitivity means the proportion of true positives correctly identified and specificity is the proportion of true negatives correctly identified.

There are additional problems, such as reproducibility of results, which is the measure of agreement between results obtained in the same subjects by different observers (inter-observer reproducibility) and by the same observers on different occasions (intra-observer reproducibility).

It will be obvious that in some fields of case-finding, there will be problems of determining whether the condition being sought is, in fact, present or not. Thus, if we were looking for social isolation or 'loneliness' as a disability, it is probable that different observers would come up with different answers. Chamberlain[16] considered these matters in relation to screening tests in the elderly. She used standard interviewing techniques and compared findings with those of objective tests. She found that screening questions related to hearing loss missed more than half of those who had a hearing loss in excess of 40 decibels in essential frequencies (500 – 2,000 c.p.s.), which was arbitrarily defined as representing significant deafness. Simple screening for visual loss (a near vision reading test and a Snellen's test at three metres) missed about 25 per cent of persons whom the ophthalmologist classed as having defective vision. In both these examples, sensitivity seemed poor. The ophthalmologist also classed as normal 30 per cent of persons whom the tester had thought to be abnormal, i.e. the specificity also was rather low and hence validity of the procedures seemed disappointing.

The problem now becomes one of trying to decide where the 'truth' really lies and this is a formidable difficulty. What, for example, is the significance of the difference in results of self-assessment of health by old people from those of a 'screening observer' or indeed from those of the 'absolute standard' of so-called objective tests? Research workers have been puzzled and discouraged by these large discrepancies, but it is possible that they are less daunting than they appear. Thus it is arguable that a detailed pathophysiological assessment is in fact less valid in screening terms in an elderly person than is perceived loss of effective function which is leading to difficulties in maintaining customary life-styles and independence. Viewed thus, the apparent precision of objective tests becomes less valid than a general assessment of functional capacity and loss with appraisal of what may be done to remedy deficiencies which arise from lost function. Thus a 20 decibel loss of hearing in important frequencies in a mentally alert old person may be fully compatible with satisfactory communication while an equal degree of hearing loss in a mentally impaired (or agitated or depressed) elderly individual could be associated with significant communication problems. More obvious are the discrepancies between objective tests of joint function (for example detailed clinical examination and X-rays) and associated functional impairment, because it is well recognised that many old persons may have marked abnormalities of knees, hips or spine and yet manage to lead full and satisfying lives while others may have considerable limitations upon life-style with much less 'objective' abnormality.

Thus, when the search is aimed at the detection of functional loss in this way, the use of objective criteria for 'normality' becomes less important and some, at least, of the discouraging lack of validity becomes less significant.

Nevertheless, formidable problems exist in devising and testing the optimum case-finding procedures and research is urgently required.

**What should be the Content of Case-finding Procedures?**

It is suggested that case-finding should be directed specially towards the disabilities which are most likely to be unreported, i.e. those shown in Figure 12.2 above. These are the disabilities associated with the locomotor system (especially the feet), bladder disturbance and mental disability (both dementia and depression). To this should be added loss of vision and hearing and perhaps impairment of postural control (as evidenced by history of falls, unsteadiness of gait, loss of confidence in going out, etc.). In addition, enquiry should be made as to diet and this may readily be condensed into a few questions covering such items as number of cooked meals per week, consumption of meat, fish, milk, cheese and eggs, plus an estimate of fruit and vegetable intake. A quick inspection by the visitor of the kitchen and the larder will often enable a reasonable estimate to be made of how accurate the old person's information may be (many may describe diets of almost Cordon Bleu excellence which are manifestly improbable when related to an empty larder or meagre cooking facilities!). How many visitors per week? How many outings per week? What is the degree of family and extra-family contact? Does the subject belong to any organised group such as a church, a lunch club or recreational group? Enquiry may be made as to accident hazards and facilities for heating in winter; in addition, an increasingly important item is that concerned with drugs. Finally, assessment of mental health must be included and this is mainly directed at the detection of dementia and depression. The Kilsyth Questionnaire[17] provides a useful example of a tried and practicable instrument of this type.

What is now urgently required is a basic 'case-finding package' of validated questions and observations. This would be of proven effectiveness as used by health visitors or others and suitable for modification to allow local needs.

## Who should Carry Out the Screening or Case-finding Procedures?

It has generally been assumed that in health matters the ideal was to have a medically qualified person to perform the required enquiry and any other individual would tend to be regarded as second-best. Whenever a 'less highly qualified' person was to be entrusted with the task, this was usually excused on the grounds that there were insufficient doctors to go round. This argument has been used against the adoption of case-finding, since general practitioners already had too much to do. Giving more thought to the problem, however, leads one to the realisation that the doctor is not necessarily the best person to perform case-finding in old age. Often the doctor's training has not equipped him well for the uncovering of multiple functional and social deficits. This may be seen by doctors as less rewarding and 'less important' than many other medical activities and thus may be performed with less interest and enthusiasm by them. It is necessary therefore to consider whether some other member of the primary care team may not be a more appropriate operator and since the necessary enquiry encompasses both health and social aspects, health visitors have often been assumed to be the most appropriate persons. There is no doubt that the health visitor's training and background in prevention and health education should equip her adequately to undertake this kind of work and many health visitors have indeed shown great interest and effectiveness in this field.[15] Some problems, however, exist, for example health visitors have been conditioned to see child welfare and maternity work as their principal sphere of action and not all of them will take an enthusiastic interest in problems at the other end of life. Health visitors also have other demands upon their time (in the fields of mental health, 'problem families', sexually transmitted diseases, accident prevention, etc.) and they may find it impossible to devote the necessary time and energy to the demanding requirements of case-finding in the elderly.

My colleagues and I, however, showed[18] that a staff nurse could be readily trained to detect with considerable accuracy important disabilities and disease states, both physical and mental. This investigation strongly suggested that any well motivated individual with general nursing training could readily be taught how to assess the important needs of elderly subjects and would obtain considerable satisfaction from the task.

My own feeling is that the formal training and educational background of the individual are probably much less important than attitude, degree of interest and motivation, and I have little doubt that many persons of good intelligence could readily be taught the techniques of speaking to old people, gaining their confidence and thus an understanding of their met and unmet needs.

It is probable that, should case-finding be proven to have high value and its practice be extended, we may have to consider the need for special 'case-finders' (perhaps they could be termed 'counsellors'?) who could be recruited from individuals of widely differing backgrounds, but all sharing a high degree of interest and motivation towards this type of work. In the present context of rising unemployment and with more jobs in the future threatened by the advent of microprocessors and related technology, is it too fanciful to suggest that this activity could provide a satisfying and worthwhile alternative to unemployment for many persons? We must certainly be prepared to consider some such arrangements in the face of steep increases in numbers of aged persons.

## Which Elderly Persons should be Screened?

In any screening programme, decisions have to be made regarding the individuals or groups of individuals to be included. Some have argued that this is a service which should be offered to all, for example the Age Concern Report of 1978.[10] Others have maintained that the public will in any case demand screening and even if 'no long term evidence exists that the course of disease is influenced by multiphasic health testing this is largely irrelevant', since it will become an expectation.[19]

My own view is that universal case-finding is neither practicable nor desirable. It would require the allocation of large resources of space, equipment and skilled manpower and until more evidence has accrued of its value and cost-effectiveness it should be resisted.

It is therefore necessary to be selective in our approach and to attempt to identify those categories of old people who are most likely to be experiencing difficulties and for whom existing services might provide significant support and relief.

I would at present suggest the following categories as being specially 'at risk' of medical and social deterioration and therefore being potential beneficiaries of case-finding measures.

(1) The very old, i.e. those age 85 or more. While age alone is not a certain predictor of disability, nevertheless the very old are more likely to be afflicted. The work of Akhtar and his colleagues[3] has already been referred to as showing that disabling conditions will be detected in about four out of five in this age group.

(2) The isolated, i.e. those living alone and separated from their families. This again must be qualified since it is well known that many old persons who live alone and have few visitors are not unhappy, appear remarkably self-sufficient and may stoutly deny loneliness. Others, by comparison, may be well visited and yet express strong feelings of loneliness and even despair. Nevertheless, an old person who is living alone with no relatives nearby is undoubtedly more liable to become isolated and withdrawn than one who is living with a spouse or who is part of an active extended family network.

(3) Those who have recently changed their dwelling. This includes

those who have moved house or who have gone into residential care as well as those who have gone to live with relatives. Old people are very sensitive to changes of environment and living arrangements and frequently react adversely. The longer an old lady has been in one setting, the deeper will be her roots and the more painful will be any uprooting process. The problems may be obvious, as in unfamiliarity with new heating or cooking arrangements, fears associated with quarterly gas or electricity bills (for someone previously accustomed to a coin-operated meter), worries about shopping from mobile (and more expensive) shops. More complex and subtle but equally dangerous problems are associated with the psychological stresses of making new friends and getting to know new neighbours. The value here of the continuity provided by a known general practitioner or health visitor can be very important.

(4) Those who have been widowed. There is a wealth of evidence to show that widowhood is associated with increased morbidity and mortality in the bereaved spouse and this is certainly borne out by clinical experience in older subjects. It is not at all surprising that the old lady who has spent her whole adult life in the service of others – first her family then her ageing husband – should become depressed and lose her sense of purpose when her husband eventually succumbs. She needs much help and support at this critical phase of her life and it is reasonable to include this category in the high-risk group and to institute special surveillance for a period of months, or even a year or two.

(5) Those who have been discharged from hospital. It is often found that the elderly are at special risk after discharge from hospital for a variety of reasons. It is probable that they suffered an illness or social crisis of considerable severity to occasion hospital admission in the first instance and with their diminished powers of recovery it is likely that they will be precariously placed for some time thereafter. At a basic level, it is possible that the essential requirements of life may be prejudiced through their absence from home, for example inadequate supplies of food and heating fuel in the home. The old person who was just managing to cope in the daily struggle of life may, after hospital admission, no longer be able to do so, and so social incapacity becomes manifest. While it may be hoped that the hospital will have foreseen all these difficulties and made suitable after care arrangements, this cannot be relied upon, especially since many old people may deliberately minimise their difficulties as a result of unrealistic wishful thinking.

## Other High-risk Groups

It is suggested that general practitioners and other members of primary care teams should make a special study of their local conditions and formulate their own registers of high-risk persons which may or may not include the above categories.

Barber and his colleagues[20] in Glasgow have experimented with a postal questionnaire sent to patients aged 70 or more in a practice list. More than four out of five of the elderly who were approached responded to the enquiry and follow-up by primary care team members showed that this system had satisfactory validity with sensitivity of 0.95 and specificity of 0.68. These workers conclude that the work in case-finding programmes could be reduced by one-fifth by the use of such a postal enquiry. In a sense this is a local attempt to get old people themselves to define their own high-risk groups. The items covered by the questionnaire embraced health and social aspects.

## What is the Value to the Individual Old Person?

This, of course, is the crucial question and also the most difficult to answer. it is obvious that case-finding by itself cannot possibly produce any betterment of the lot of the screened individual. Thus, an old lady who is experiencing difficulty in getting about and in accomplishing the things she wishes to do on account of stiff and painful knees will not be one whit better for having a doctor (or health visitor) examine her, perhaps arrange X-rays of knees and pronounce that she has osteoarthritis! It is important therefore that the conditions sought should be those for which there is a prospect of cure, alleviation or rehabilitation, or failing all these that there should be services to meet the needs of the individual who is disabled in this way. Thus adequate social and rehabilitation services must be available without undue delay. With the development of day centres, day hospitals, home help services, lunch clubs and home meals services these requirements are being more adequately fulfilled, so that case-finding becomes more justifiable and rational than in the past. It is, however, essential that estimates of increased demands which are likely to arise from case-finding programmes should be made in advance, otherwise the result is likely to be wasted effort plus frustration and disappointment.

One important aspect of assessment of the effectiveness of case-finding measures which is usually neglected is their effect upon morale, and Luker[21] has proposed the use of a life satisfaction index. She has shown that this fairly simple index may be successfully used with elderly Scottish women and it seems reasonable to suggest that this type of evaluation should be incorporated in any assessment of case-finding measures.

## What is the Cost-effectiveness of this Procedure and what Priority should it be Accorded in the Provision of Health Services?

The customary method of gauging effectiveness of a health care programme is to compare the outcome in test subjects with matched controls and for case-finding schemes the criteria to be studied would include morbidity, mortality and use of resources (plus assessment of life satisfaction as noted above). Test subjects and controls would have to be followed up for a period of two or three years (as in the South-East London Screening Study already referred to) and strictly random allocation ensured. The complexities are likely to be greater in older subjects, since the objectives of case-finding are less clear than in younger subjects who are being screened for such relatively clear-cut conditions as, say, hypertension or carcinoma of cervix *in situ*. Thus a reduction in mortality in 85-year-old subjects would not necessarily be a primary objective, since it is unlikely that the discovery of unmet needs in this group would lead to prolongation of life. Rather, it might be hoped that the elderly individual would be enabled to remain independent for longer and derive greater satisfaction thereby. At the same time it might be hoped that cost to the community would be reduced. It is especially desirable that the need for institutional care should be postponed or avoided or required for shorter periods, for example for a specific purpose of rehabilitation or for a brief respite for supporting family members. The consequence of any significant reduction in demand for institutional care would inevitably be an increased need for community services, for example day care, home help and home nursing services. It is therefore essential that those who plan case-finding procedures in the elderly should consult in advance with those who are responsible for the provision of community services.

As regards the cost-effectiveness of case-finding in old age, we possess little or no knowledge upon which to base conclusions and hence we are not in a position to assess the priority which ought to be accorded to such measures. Despite this, my strongest impression after twenty years in this field is that the greatest hope for containing the demands of an ageing population lies in the field of preventive care.

The greatest urgency now is for properly conducted scientific trials of case-finding and I suggest that this would encompass the following:

(1) the evolution of a practicable case-finding 'package' – what questions to ask and what observations to make;
(2) trials of this validated 'package' in different high-risk groups of old people by different kinds of observers; and
(3) finally a controlled trial of the validated case-finding procedure with outcome assessed in terms of morbidity, dependency, use of services (especially of institutional services) and life satisfaction.

## Conclusion

Mankind has never before had to cope with so rapidly increasing a number of ageing individuals, as more and more realise their full potential life span. New methods for maintaining this must be tried and if found effective, introduced widely. Case-finding seems likely to have great possibilities for improving the health and happiness of old people and it is a matter of urgency to determine whether it is an effective preventive measure and how it may best be applied.

## References.

1. Williamson, J., Stokoe, I.H., Gray, S., Fisher, M., and Smith, A. (1964) 'Old People at Home: Their Unreported Needs', *Lancet, 1*, 1117-20
2. Andrews, G.R., Cowan, N.R., and Anderson, W.F. (1971) in G. MacLachlan (ed.), *Problems and Progress in Medical Care*, Nuffield Provincial Hospitals Trust, Oxford University Press, Oxford
3. Akhtar, A.J., Broe, G.A., Crombie, Agnes, McLean, W.M.R., Andrews, G.R., and Caird, F.I. (1973) 'Disability and Dependence in the Elderly at Home', *Age and Ageing, 2*, 102-11
4. Thomas, P. (1968) 'Experiences of Two Preventive Clinics for the Elderly', *British Medical Journal, 2*, 357-60
5. Burns, C. (1969) 'Geriatric Care in General Practice', *J. Roy. Coll. Gen. Pract., 18*, 289-96
6. Currie, G., MacNeill, R.M., Walker, J.G., Barnie, Elva, and Mudie, Elizabeth W. (1974) 'Medical and Social Screening of Patients aged 70 to 72 by an Urban General Practice Health Team', *British Medical Journal, 2*, 108-11
7. Barber, J.H., and Wallis, Joan B. (1976) 'Assessment of the Elderly in General Practice', *J. Roy. Coll. Gen. Pract., 26*, 106-14
8. Lowther, C.P., MacLeod, R.D.M., and Williamson, J. (1970) 'Evaluation of Early Diagnostic Services for the Elderly', *British Medical Journal, 3*, 275-7

9. Williams, I. (1974) 'A Follow-up of Geriatric Patients after Social Medical Assessments', *J. Roy. Coll. Gen. Pract., 24*, 341-6
10. *The National Policy* (1978) Age Concern Report
11. *Prevention and Health* (1977) Cmnd, 7047, HMSO, London
12. Editorial (1978) *Lancet, 1*, 54
13. Cutler, J., Ramcharan, E., Felman, R., Siegelaub, A.B., Campbell, C., Friedman, G.D., Dales, L.G., and Collen, M.F. (1973) 'Multiphasic Check-up Evaluation Study, 1-3', *Preventive Medicine, 2*, 197
14. The South-East London Screening Study Group (1977) 'A Controlled Trial of Multiphasic Screening in Middle-Age: Results of the South-east London Screening Study', *Int. J. Epidem., 6*, 357-63
15. Williamson, J. (1967) 'Detecting Disease in Clinical Geriatrics', *Gerontol. Clin., 9*, 236-42
16. Chamberlain, J.O.P.(1973) 'Screening Elderly People', *Proc. Roy. Soc. Med., 66*, 888-9
17. Powell, C., and Crombie, Agnes (1974) 'The Kilsyth Questionnaire: a Method of Screening Elderly People at Home', *Age and Ageing, 3*, 23-8
18. Milne, J.S., Maule, M.M., Cormack, S., and Williamson, J. (1972) 'The Design and Testing of a Questionnaire and Examination to Assess Physical and Mental Health in Older People Using a Staff Nurse as the Observer', *J. Chron. Dis., 25*, 385-405
19. Garfield, S.R. (1970) 'Multiphasic Health Testing and Medical Care as a Right', *New Engl. J. Med., 283*, 1087-9
20. Barber, J.H., Wallis, Joan B., and McKeating, Edith (1978) 'A Postal Screening Questionnaire in Preventive Geriatric Care' (personal communication)
21. Luker, Karen A. (1979) 'Measuring Life Satisfaction in an Elderly Female Population', *J. Advanced Nursing, 4*, 503-11

# 13 SERVICE INNOVATIONS IN GERIATRIC PSYCHIATRY

Kenneth Shulman

## Introduction

Health services for the elderly, and old age psychiatric services in particular, have predictable frustrations. Almost everywhere, their value and the need for them is acknowledged, but financial and territorial considerations regularly impede their implementation. Geriatric psychiatry is a 'Johnny Come Lately' in the history of health services and every 'new boy' faces the problem of cracking the barriers of the establishment and changing long-standing practices and modes of thinking.

Out of necessity and often within severe limitations there have evolved a variety of innovative ways in which psychiatric services are provided. These innovations are dependent, of course, on a number of variables, which have been reviewed by Arie and Isaacs.[1] These include the available facilities, the personality, interests and philosophy of the 'main driving force', usually a psychiatrist or a geriatrician, as well as the nature and needs of the population being served. I would include among these factors the broader social system and philosophy of health care within a particular country. This ranges from the National Health Service of the United Kingdom, through the modified form of universal health care available in a country like Canada, to the predominantly private health care scheme of the United States. In this latter system, financial restrictions on the amount of billing allowed in a given period of time may influence the treatment available for an individual elderly patient. This would not be a consideration, for example, in the United Kingdom or Canada.

The variety of different types of services and innovative programmes that have evolved have been well described in the Joint Information Service report of the APA[2] and in other reports.[1,3,4] Individual reports of other innovative services include notable contributions by Robinson,[5] Arie,[6] Baker,[7] Whitehead,[8] Godber[9] and Pitt.[10] Different models have been proposed, but a consensus about issues and aims seems to be emerging. These include:

(1) an emphasis on community care and deinstitutionalisation –

the elderly are usually happier within their own homes and it is desirable to support them there;
(2) services should tackle the full range of psychiatric disorder seen in the elderly;
(3) a multi-disciplinary approach is necessary, with collaboration with a geriatric medical service in order to be able to provide a comprehensive service for the elderly with multiple problems.

The following description of the first year's experience in developing a psychiatric service for the elderly, in Toronto, Canada, illustrates many of the problems and issues mentioned above. This will be a largely personal account that reflects this author's own biases and philosophy towards health care of the elderly and is not meant to be a comprehensive review. This report will emphasise the specific innovations that have been developed as a result of the particular circumstances of available facilities, personnel and established patterns of health care within this setting.

## The Facility

I decided upon a general hospital setting (Sunnybrook Medical Centre) in which to develop a new psychiatric service for the elderly. The new geriatric service was to be integrated within the Department of Psychiatry and was accepted as a fully fledged section of the department. It was felt to be important that the geriatric service was not isolated or viewed somehow as outside the sphere of a highly valued Department of Psychiatry. In addition, another attraction was that a geriatrician, also trained in the United Kingdom, was already in the hospital and had been administering a section of the hospital mainly caring for chronic patients for the Department of Veterans Affairs.

It is my conviction that the psychiatry of old age can flourish best within the environment of a general hospital wherever feasible. It is not necessary to emphasise the very high prevalence of physical illnesses found among elderly psychiatric patients. The very close association of physical and mental disorders among the elderly has been shown time and time again.[11,12,13] Consequently, a great deal of anxiety and conflict over the physical care of the elderly can be generated in a psychiatric unit. However, within the setting of a general hospital this anxiety is dispelled to a great extent when one operates with the security of 24-hour coverage and where consultations from a wide variety of medical and surgical services are readily available. The potential for collaborating with a geriatrician was a great attraction and will be dealt with in a later section.

The restrictions under which this new service was to develop, however, were significant. Ten beds were assigned in the general psychiatric ward for the elderly. No additional staff were available and it was necessary, therefore, to carve out of the existing resources a cohesive and comprehensive unit that previously had been delivering services to the elderly in a fragmentary fashion.

## Staffing Issues

Morale problems among the staff have been addressed by Arie,[13] Clarke[14] and in some of the Committees of Inquiry of the late sixties and early seventies in the United Kingdom.[15,16] Again these problems are dependent upon the setting and type of unit in which the service is to be developed. The issues in the setting in which I work are different from those in long-stay wards and large mental hospitals where other geriatric services have evolved. In a teaching hospital that viewed itself as giving 'acute care' within a 'therapeutic milieu' there were special problems. The imminent development of a geriatric service within a general psychiatric ward created a great deal of anxiety among the nursing staff. The fantasy that there would be a group of decrepit, difficult, elderly patients who were 'placement problems' challenged their roles and identities as 'therapists'. This was true of other disciplines, including social work, occupational therapy, psychology and the psychiatric trainees themselves.

On a mixed adult ward and in a general department of psychiatry, it was essential to establish a 'team' that was to work closely with the elderly. Without such a 'team' there is the danger that the staff who merely rotate through the service would not have the desired sense of purpose and commitment and this in turn would lead to major morale problems. Fortunately, five nurses volunteered to be assigned full-time to the geriatric service and, with time, an occupational therapist, social worker and public health (community) nurse were added. One general psychiatric resident was assigned full-time to the ten-bed unit. All members of the team saw themselves as providing an important and worthwhile service and, indeed, felt that they were working together for the benefit of the patient.

From what I have observed in the United Kingdom, there are two basic ingredients necessary for a geriatric service to flourish – the generation of enthusiasm and a sense of purpose to the unit. The nature of work in this area is such that the staff require regular booster injections of morale and close monitoring of the level of gratification from their work. Regular team meetings and in-service education have helped in this regard.

In a multi-disciplinary approach, it is important to establish a division of labour based on the particular expertise of each member of the team. However, depending on the personality, drive and abilities of individual team members, some flexibility and blurring of roles must occur in order to maximise the skills available. Hence, in our own team a very capable occupational therapist participated in home visits and community follow-up and became a much more prominent team member than has been traditional for occupational therapists.

## Comprehensive Services

One of the aims of the geriatric service was to provide care for the full range of psychiatric disorders. In addition, it was important to provide as comprehensive a service as possible without fragmenting the care of the elderly mentally disordered individual.

Essentially, there are three types of patients in a geriatric psychiatry service. First are the functionally ill elderly who are relatively well physically. Second, there are the functionally ill elderly, who have concomitant serious physical problems; and third, there are the ambulatory cognitively impaired patients who may or may not have serious physical disorders. As my initial mandate for in-patients included only a ten-bed unit on a mixed general psychiatry ward, I was forced to make some modifications in the kind of patients that one could readily treat in such a setting. In particular, it became apparent fairly early on that the demented patient was not treated readily in a mixed setting such as this and required special services and facilities within the hospital. More importantly, an effective community support system and day hospital facility is necessary if the unit is to function as both an assessment and a relief unit. This is now a major restriction under which we are operating, but we are moving towards organising a collaborative effort with geriatric medicine, family practice and rehabilitation medicine to develop a special 'joint psychogeriatric service' on the medical ward. Here we should be able to treat a wide variety of patients whose most prominent or major disability is cognitive impairment and further develop our community services.

Surprisingly, for me there has been relatively little demand for the assessment or management of demented patients. This is largely due to two factors. The proportion of over-65s in Canada is running at somewhat less than 10 per cent,[17] compared to over 14 per cent in the United Kingdom. This demographic difference is particularly apparent in the 80-and-over age group. This population trend will change dramatically within the next twenty years, when the 80-and-over population in Canada will double.

Another major factor is the traditionally poor service given by psychiatrists to the demented, as most psychiatrists have never viewed this population as within their sphere of responsibility or interest. Patients suffering from dementia have been dealt with largely by social services in nursing home settings. Consequently, the vast majority of referrals to a new psychiatrist with a special interest in the elderly have been for the management of the functionally ill or for the assessment of diagnostic problems where cognitive impairment is questionable. I hope that as the service develops and we are better able to deal effectively with the demented, we will encourage more referrals for this group.

My own view is that there is a need for different treatment for the cognitively impaired elderly compared to the functionally ill. Treatment effort and orientation, too, are quite different for staff dealing with the demented and the functionally ill. Again in terms of staff morale, it is important to ensure that one is meeting the needs of the care-takers. In addition, for the functionally ill patient who is *compos mentis*, it is particularly stressful to be placed in the same living quarters with significantly demented patients. This seems to be an unnecessary obstacle to recovery if it is at all possible to establish differential treatment facilities for these two groups.

### Assessment

Availability is the essence of all psychiatric services to the elderly. It is of no value to have an excellent assessment procedure if there is a long waiting list. Various innovations are required in order to have time to defuse a crisis or provide rapid intervention while performing non-urgent assessments.

Arie[6] has proposed a model by which the home visit is the fundamental tool for all assessments. This has proved to be the most effective way to gain a grasp of the problem and plan management. In addition, the assessment at home can prevent unnecessary admissions to hospital that may complicate the clinical picture and course. In light of time restrictions and limited manpower, I have adopted a modified form of this approach in our own setting. When referrals are made to our service, an initial screen identifies those patients where cognitive impairment is the predominant problem as well as those patients who are unable or unwilling to come to the hospital for an assessment. That is, the functionally ill or depressed patient is seen in the office, whereas the patient with cerebral organic disorder is seen in his own setting. While this may be less than ideal, I have found this to be a reasonable method of determining how the initial assessment needs to be done, Ideally, the home assessment should be a joint effort, with a social worker or occupational therapist when appropriate, and a psychiatrist.

The weekly schedule of the psychiatrist dealing with the elderly must be flexible and it is far too easy to fill up a busy week and simply leave no time for 'urgent assessments'. Otherwise the Emergency Department acts as the 'safety valve', and it is known to handle poorly and often inappropriately the psychogeriatric cases that come its way. Families who end up pleading for admission are viewed incorrectly as 'dumping or sloughing' their elderly family members. In effect, they are demonstrating the result of an ineffective community assessment system.

## Geriatrician-Psychiatrist Collaboration

Collaboration with geriatric medicine is becoming more and more a fundamental aspect of health care for the elderly.[18,19] The main purpose of this collaboration is twofold:

(1) to prevent the elderly patient falling between the two stools of geriatric medicine and geriatric psychiatry and thereby reducing conflict, anxiety and frustration;
(2) collaboration results in reciprocal consultation and mutual benefit.

In our own unit, we are fortunate in having a senior resident in geriatric medicine as our regular consultant to the in-patient service. We note that when medical or surgical residents are asked to come to see elderly patients, it is often difficult for them to motivate themselves to take the consultation in a serious vein. On the other hand, a specialist in geriatric medicine seems to be able to relate much better to our geriatric team, generating a much greater level of enthusiasm and hopefulness towards therapeutic outcome. Consequently, the geriatric resident has become in effect a member of our team. While attending our weekly case conference, he has an opportunity to learn psychiatry and also contribute to discussion with particular emphasis on the physical factors that are relevant in any one case. This type of close collaboration is possible only within a general hospital that has both a geriatrician and a psychogeriatrician on the premises. The great effect on morale and actual service to the patient has become evident in our brief experiment in this kind of collaborative effort.

**Follow-up Clinic**

A major problem among the elderly is the recurrent and chronic nature of functional disorders.[20,21] Close follow-up is an essential part of the management of functional disorders in old age. This is a difficult task in a high-risk group of patients who have multiple problems. Consequently, a major innovation at Sunnybrook Medical Centre has been the development of a multi-disciplinary follow-up clinic where we follow all patients who have been discharged from the in-patient unit. That is, we are dealing with the more seriously disordered and perhaps the more fragile and vulnerable population of a psychiatric service. Because this is an open clinic to which patients are given appointments, it lends itself more to the treatment of the functionally disordered and is really not appropriate for the management of dementia. Within the clinic, in addition to the psychiatrist, two out-patient nurses, an occupational therapist and a social worker are present. The clinic is open in the sense that despite the fact that appointments are given, the patients are given the clear message that they can 'drop in' if necessary. The atmosphere is informal as patients meet together with the various workers in the clinic while the psychiatrist sees them individually for a brief period. The concept of an open clinic has been distressing to some centres where fears of abuse of this opportunity are prominent. However, it has been our experience that in reality no patient has 'abused' the system and the few patients who have come earlier than the appointed date have done so for very valid reasons and have often prevented full-blown relapses.

With the availability of a multi-disciplinary team, it is possible to review a large number of patients in a morning. The psychiatrist in such a setting can restrict his assessments to evaluations of mental state and review of ongoing therapies, while the other members of the team can address particular issues that relate to their own speciality and to their own expertise within the community. In addition, the organisation and collation of various investigations, appointments and reports are done much more readily within this kind of team setting. We are thus able to maintain the close follow-up necessary for many of these patients with the aim of preventing relapses that are so common among this group of patients. There is the added benefit of allowing workers on the in-patient unit to see patients who are doing well and functioning in the community. This is yet another morale factor, as the in-patient unit sees the most disturbed, refractory and chronic patients.

**Community Workers**

As staff in the hospital have been limited in their availability for community work, we have had to utilise the existing community resources, including public health nurses and a group of occupational therapists who work in the community. A liaison with these organisations has been an effective way of dealing with many of our patients who require follow-up assessment at home. In return for these services we have offered consultation for problems these workers are facing with patients referred from other agencies. In addition, we have established a continuing teaching programme for these community workers. This hospital-based programme has given mutual benefit and illustrates the type of arrangement that can be helpful when personnel are limited.

A unique problem facing us in North America is the lack of a catchment area for most general hospitals. Where no defined population is assigned to any one setting, this creates major problems and we are in the process of attempting to establish independently a catchment area to identify the patients for whom we in our unit will be responsible. This should illustrate how much more efficient health care planning and evaluation can be when one's area of responsibility is clearly defined.

**Education and Research**

In an academic setting this is a very important area that also can add to the morale and sense of purpose described above. We are hoping that we can develop a unit that can provide both an exemplary service on a small scale and incorporate an active research and training programme at the same time. A psychogeriatric service can be the base for many disciplines that are involved in the health care of the elderly and will, we hope, be used as a training ground for both general psychiatrists and for specialists in geriatric psychiatry as well as other disciplines such as social work, occupational therapy and psychology.

For those services that are beginning within an academic setting, it is extremely important that one's efforts are documented, evaluated and reported as widely as possible, so that the greatest benefit can accrue from innovations that are tried within particular settings. Especially in the area of geriatric psychiatry, which is such a new speciality and where a multiplicity of approaches is prevalent, the type of research and evaluation noted above is extremely important. The opportunity to train many disciplines is valuable and I believe most useful within the hospital-based setting.

My experience in this field also reflects a new stage in the development of geriatric psychiatry. Until very recently, there had been no formal training in geriatric psychiatry and psychiatrists have become involved more out of their own interest or by necessity. Moreover, experience alone was their teacher and the pioneers in this field learned by doing. I had the benefit of specialised training and returned to a setting in which this experience was valued. Thus, a favourable atmosphere had been created for the development of a new psychiatric service for the elderly and that represents a distinct change from the conditions in which psychiatrists and geriatricians have had to operate until recently.

## References

1. Arie, T., and Isaacs, A.D. (1977) 'The Development of Psychiatric Services for the Elderly in Britain' in F. Post and A.D. Isaacs (eds.), *Studies in Geriatric Psychiatry*, John Wiley, Chichester
2. Glasscote, R.M., Gudeman, J.E., and Miles, D.G. (1977) *Creative Mental Health Services for the Elderly*, Joint Information Service, American Psychiatric Association, Washington, DC
3. Jolley, D.J., and Arie, T. (1978) 'Organisation of Psychogeriatric Services', *British Journal of Psychiatry, 132*, 1-11
4. Pitt, B. (1980) 'Growing Points in the Psychiatry of Old Age. Organisation of Services', *Canadian Journal of Psychiatry, 25*, 15-25
5. Robinson, R.A. (1962) 'The Practice of a Psychiatric Geriatric Unit', *Gerontologia Clinica,* Suppl., 1-19
6. Arie, T. (1970) 'The First Year of the Goodmayes Psychiatric Service for Old

People', *Lancet, ii*, 1179-82
7. Baker, A.A. (1974) 'Why psychogeriatrics?' *Lancet, i*, 795-6
8. Whitehead, J.A. (1972) 'Services for Old People with Mental Symptoms', *Community Health*, 83-6
9. Godber, C. (1976) 'The Psychiatry of Old Age' in J.T. Leeming (ed.), *Doctors and Old Age*, London, British Geriatrics Society
10. Pitt, B. (1974) *Psychogeriatrics*, Churchill Livingstone, Edinburgh and London
11. Kay, D.W.K., and Bergmann, K. (1966) 'Physical Disability and Mental Health in Old Age', *Journal of Psychosomatic Research, 10*, 3-12
12. Eastwood, M.R., and Trevelyan, M.H. (1972) 'Relationship between Physical and Psychiatric Disorder', *Psychological Medicine, 2*, 363-72
13. Arie, T. (1971) 'Morale and the Planning of Psychogeriatric Services', *British Medical Journal, 3*, 166-70
14. Clarke, M. (1974) *The Care of Patients on a Long Stay Psychogeriatric Ward and Working with Elderly Patients: Nurses Expectations and Experiences,* research reports to DHSS
15. *Report of Inquiry on Allegations of Ill Treatment of Patients and Other Irregular Activites at the Ely Hospital, Cardiff* (1969) Comnd. 3975, HMSO, London
16. *Report of the Committee of Inquiry into Whittingham Hospital* (1972) Comnd. 4861, National Health Service, HMSO, London
17. Statistics Canada (1979) *Canada's Elderly*, Ministry of Supply and Service, Ottawa
18. Arie, T., and Dunn, T. (1973) 'A "Do-it-yourself" Psychiatric-geriatric Unit', *Lancet, ii*, 313-16
19. Pitt, B., and Silver, C.P. (1980) 'The Combined Approach to Geriatrics and Psychiatry. Evaluation of a Joint Unit in a Teaching Hospital District', *Age and Ageing, 9*, 33-7
20. Post, F. (1972) 'The Management and Nature of Depressive Illness in Late Life: a Follow-through Study', *British Journal of Psychiatry, 121*, 393-404
21. Post, F. (1978) 'The Functional Psychoses' in Isaacs and Post, *Studies in Geriatric Psychiatry*

# 14 IS GERIATRICS A SPECIALTY?

Bernard Isaacs

How this question is answered is predictable from who is asked. General physicians (internists) deny that geriatric medicine needs special skills, but claim that they possess these. Geriatricians are certain that they are specialists, but uncertain about what they are specialists in.

I believe that geriatric medicine is potentially a specialty of the highest order. Unhappily, its scope has been debased by preoccupation with health-care economics; and its grandeur has been obscured by relegation and rejection.

In this chapter, I shall endeavour to rehabilitate geriatrics. I shall trace the history of geriatric medicine in the United Kingdom, describe its present status and discuss its immediate prospects. I shall mention alternative models of practice; and conclude with a roseate vision of a desirable future.

## The History of Geriatric Medicine in the United Kingdom

British geriatrics, like many other bastards, was born in the Poor House. It was fathered by neglect and nurtured by necessity, until it grew into a great ungainly monster; and now it is about to be married off to General Medicine.

### *The Birth and Parentage of British Geriatrics*

Half a generation ago Britain was in the Dark Ages in regard to the public and private care of the indigent elderly sick. Many hospitals, especially the teaching hospitals, exercised positive discrimination against the elderly. House physicians of my day were instructed to repel all applicants for admission if they were over the age of 65 on the unarguable grounds that 'We don't take that type of patient in here.' The general practitioner could be unpleasant about this at times, but his invisible reproaches were much to be preferred to the wrath of the Chief next morning when he found one of 'his' beds put to such inappropriate use. Thus these good and famous men, our teachers, transmitted to us, their students, their blind rejection of the elderly. On reflection it is difficult to discern what they feared. By excluding ill old people from teaching hospitals, they excluded the study of ill old people from medical science and the knowledge of ill old people from the future leaders of the medical and nursing professions. The wealthy elderly ill took solace in nursing homes, private nurses and bath chairs in the park. As for the poor . . . 'There were places for them,' in the telling phrase of the day.

What these 'places' were only came to my knowledge after qualification, when I was led into a former Poor House by my mentor, who subsequently became Britain's first professor of geriatric medicine. An unbelievable sight it was too: our present doctors in training think that I and my peers exaggerate when we talk of the day rooms, unheated save by a great iron stove discharging yellow smoke; unfurnished save by wooden kitchen chairs; and peopled with upwards of sixty old men, dressed in calico nightshirts of umbilical length and coarse cloth jackets and trousers, urinating on the floor beneath them, and countering the odour with that of indifferent tobacco. Pipe-smoking was the only occupational therapy provided – the pipes lighted by the attendant, for the ownership of matches was forbidden. The patients left in bed in the cheerless ward were so distorted by contractures that their only human resemblance was to the foetus in the womb. They were there because they were ill, old and poor. They were there because, when the general practitioner telephoned the teaching hospital, he was told, 'Try elsewhere.' I did not like the sight of 'elsewhere'.

It was out of this Sin that geriatrics was conceived. The qualification required of its practitioners was only a determination to expel Evil. Little specialised knowledge was required: just dogged persistence, improvisation, innovation, pressure, exploitation, the refusal to accept defeat; and above all the conjunction with others of like mind, irrespective of professional affiliation.

### *The Growth and Development of British Geriatrics*

From such origins as these British geriatric medicine has developed into a large and rather splendid organisation. Departments of geriatric medicine, properly organised and staffed, are to be found throughout the United Kingdom. There is local diversity, but acceptance of common principles. All geriatricians aspire to provide their patients with the same standards of excellence that are accorded to patients of any other age group. Accurate diagnosis, comprehensive assessment, personalised treatment, appropriate rehabilitation, comprehension of the social situation and the fine tuning of resources to abilities; these are the universal aims of geriatricians. To meet these complex needs a network of services has developed, with great use of innovation and improvisation. Much of the expertise of the geriatric physician comes from the recognition of recurring patterns of disability, the interaction between physical, mental and social factors; the intelligent and flexible use of the pool of resources; and the maintenance of mutual understanding between the many professional groups involved. To understand and to control all this requires much training and experience; and your mature geriatrician is master of many skills.

And yet this rapid and substantial metamorphosis is not enough. Such indicators as we have of the value attached to the various specialities – and these include the career preferences of young graduates[1] and the allocation of merit awards[2] – places geriatric medicine at the bottom of the scale. A very high proportion of the doctors training to be future consultants in geriatric medicine in the United Kingdom were not educated in that country. The geriatrician's claim that his subject is a speciality as demanding and as rewarding as any other is denied by the career choices, if not by the words, of the young British graduate.

But what has been happening to general medicine meanwhile?

## The Growth and Development of General Medicine

While geriatrics was struggling to break out of the Poor House, the volcanic mountains of specialised scientific knowledge were erupting forth new techniques, new instruments, new needs. In order to look at a heart, a lung or a kidney properly, doctors now needed prolonged training, elaborate equipment, a large team. The future specialists were familiarised with the methods and equipment, and trained – but for what? There were not enough jobs, and highly trained men could hardly be expected to work without equipment. As has often happened before in medicine, the best became the enemy of the good. British inventiveness provided a solution by offering posts of consultant physician 'with an interest in' the appropriate speciality. The new consultant found that his 'interest' was often confined to running a weekly out-patient clinic; but as a consultant physician he took his full share of the 'acute take'. In the meantime demography and medical attitudes had been changing; and the 'acute take' cast up on the consultant's stretch of the beach very little treasure trove in relation to his own speciality but a great deal of the flotsam and jetsam of old age. The consultant physician with a special interest became the consultant physician with a special frustration. To their credit the vast majority of physicians worked hard and well in caring for their elderly acute patients, while at the same time developing their speciality interests as best they could within the resource constraints of modern British medicine. But the effect was to look for more and more help from geriatricians in order to free more and more highly valued 'acute' beds,[3] and thus the role of the geriatric physician was devalued by equating him with the 'clinical undertaker'.[4] This process was cyclical. Role devaluation diminished recruitment, impaired the efficiency of geriatric services and compounded the problem of the general and specialist physicians.

## The Marriage of British Geriatrics

At this stage the Royal College of Physicians stepped in with its analysis that the problem of providing a specialist service for the elderly was largely one of recruitment; and the best chance of stimulating recruitmet was to promote a marriage between general (internal) medicine and geriatrics.

The forthcoming marriage was first announced in the gossip columns of *The Lancet.*[5] One might easily have missed it, since the authors favoured the word 'integration', but the intention was clear. In the true style of marriage brokers it was considered that the advantages of the union to bride and groom, i.e. geriatrician and general physician, were so self-evident as not to necessitate such trifles as obtaining the prior consent of the parties or arranging the details of the marriage contract. From the conjunction of bride and groom was to spring a 'consultant physician with an interest in geriatric medicine', under whose auspices the union of the two professions would be finally and harmoniously consummated.

The Royal College of Physicians' recommendation is one of several models under continuing scrutiny. In some areas it works, in the sense that able people have been attracted to suitably planned posts, and have given of their time fairly and equally to the demands of acute hospital medical practice and to the development of hospital and community-based services for the elderly. In other areas attempts to introduce this system have failed, because the established demands on and resources of the Health Service cannot be bent into this new pattern without serious stresses; but this development will at least attract continuing interest.

An alternative pattern[6] is the age-related division of services, in which all 'medical' emergencies under an arbitrary age are accepted into the general medical service, and all over that age into the parallel geriatric service. Such an arrangement can be criticised on grounds of illogicality, segregation, ageism, duplication – but it succeeds. The medical and geriatric teams work flexibly together, interchanging patients and ideas. There are no boundary zones where responsibility is dubious, and the general practitioners receive an instant and unambiguous service. But again there have been few successful duplications of this system, largely because the unsuitable location and inadequate resources of many geriatric units make hazardous the emergency admission of large numbers of acutely ill old people.

British departments of geriatric medicine vary in their organisation, but most embody, formally or informally, some features of an age-related service, in that a varying proportion of their admissions are of very old people with the recent onset of an episode of life-threatening illness, often appearing against a background of previous disability or social deprivation, and providing the opportunity for exercising both the diagnostic and therapeutic skills of 'acute medicine' and the multidisciplinary assessment, physical, psychological and social rehabilitation and continuing hospital and community care which characterise the geriatrician's approach.

British geriatricians have been promised that a high proportion of their resources will be located in general hospitals,[7] a prerequisite for the practice of good emergency medicine for old people and satisfactory junior staff recruitment and training. But preoccupation with this highly desirable objective does not absolve the geriatrician from his responsibility for providing, organising and collaborating with a wide range of hospital and domiciliary services in meeting the total health needs of an ageing community.

I do not believe that we can or should do without the 'geriatrician' as he has developed in the United Kingdom in the past 25 years. Indeed, I believe we should encourage a separate development, because general physicians and geriatricians are like bookends; they come out of the same mould; they perform the same task; neither can manage without the other; but they face in opposite directions; and when they cease to do so what they are supporting falls down.

## The Future of British Geriatrics

I called geriatrics a bastard because it did not know who its father was.

It has behaved as if its father was Need and it has played the role of Provider. It has done the job well but has received little thanks. But I believe that the parentage of geriatric medicine is something altogether more respectable. The unique demographic feature to which geriatric medicine is the response is the survival of large numbers of people into advanced old age, for the first time in human history. The medical and social problems of human ageing have never before been so freely available for scientific study, but as yet the surface has barely been skimmed. The many academic departments of geriatric medicine now flourishing in the United Kingdom owe their existence not to the growth of scientific knowledge but to the demand that 'something be done'. Geriatric medicine has concerned itself until now primarily with *managing*. It must turn its attention to *man ageing*.

## Geriatrics: The Study of Human Ageing

Man does not age in a test tube but in an eventful world. The processes of his ageing are the interaction between the physical changes in his body, the psychological changes in his mind and the social changes in his environment. Geriatrics, not gerontology, affords the true stage for the study of human ageing. The clinician attempting to restore purpose and vitality to the life of his aged patient best perceives the oneness and the multiplicity of human ageing.

Geriatrics is the medicine of dependency, of pre-death, of the Survival of the Unfittest.[8]

## The Giants of Geriatrics

The causes of failing function in late old age are accumulation of lesions, impairment of adaptation and impoverishment of environment. These acquire medical expression in a limited number of ways, of which the most characteristic and most visible manifestations are those four great giants of geriatrics[9] – immobility, instability, incontinence and intellectual impairment.

### *Immobility*

Immobility in old age may be due to respiratory, cardiac or peripheral vascular disorders, when it is energetically investigated and treated; or to diseases of the muscles, joints or nervous system, when investigation tends to be less intensive, treatment less accurately defined and publication of results less frequent.

The geriatrician, like the general physician, pursues the causes of immobility, but views it, however caused, in terms of restriction of life-space. Draw concentric circles with radiuses respectively of 1, 5, 10, 100, 1,000 metres and your bed at the centre; and inscribe in each circle the activities you undertake, the time you spend and the values you attach. Now do the same for a prisoner in goal, a lion in a cage, a potato plant in the garden. It is thus that the geriatrician seeks to understand what immobility is. So, he may comprehend what his patient means when he describes himself as 'a prisoner in my own house'. So, he may understand the value of a treatment, however empirical, which extends life-space; and the futility of one which does not.

The geriatrician, accustomed to making house calls, or domiciliary assessment visits as he calls them, knows that the front door of the housebound sprouts locks, bolts, chains, catches and spy-holes. It has ceased to be an object for letting the insider out; it is being transposed into one for preventing the outsider from coming in. It symbolises the secondary change which will prove a secondary challenge to rehabilitation. The prisoner has come to love his chains.

Techniques for rehabilitating the house-imprisoned must be as ingenious as those required for the recidivist. For example, in an attempt to inspire a resistive old lady to walk again, a clinical psychologist, working in a geriatric unit, suggested the use of 'Green Shield' stamps, normally issued as a bonus for purchases in supermarkets. One of these was to be awarded for every yard walked each day, and they were to be stuck in a book, eventually to be exchanged for desirable consumer goods. The psychologist's insight was just right. The urge to acquire these symbols of opulence overcame the fear of venturing forth. There is much scope for extending this approach.

*Instability*

Many an old lady comes into hospital as an emergency having been found lying on the floor at home unable to rise. If in the course of falling she succeeds in breaking a bone, she can legitimately claim a ticket of admission to hospital, with the label of fractured femur. If she fails to break a bone, she arrives at hospital with no identity. If there is no one else at home, she may get in on the strength of having a 'social problem', although she might be better advised to have pneumonia or hypothermia to legitimise her admission. Lacking such credentials, she may well be sent home where she will be expected to 'cope'. What she has to cope with and how she performs this action is left undefined; but failure to do so is as much a moral as a social failure.

The real queston is 'Why did the patient fall in the first instance?' Man took millions of phylogenetic and several ontogenetic years to acquire an upright posture, yet it can be lost in an instant. Falls vary from momentary aberrations of no continuing significance to severe and permanent disruptions of the intricate neuromuscular mechanisms underlying the complex act of locomotion. This has been studied more assiduously by the practitioners of sports medicine than by the practitioners of geriatric medicine. The transport of sodium ions across cell membranes has attracted more medical interest than the transport of human beings across rooms. The balance between anion and cation absorbs many more shelf-miles of medical literature than the balance between right foot and left foot. We now know a great deal about the forces which act on joints[10] and are beginning to understand the forces that act on the minds of those who have fallen, causing loss of faith in their own stability and lack of progress in their own rehabilitation. The subject is just beginning to develop[11,12] and further progress must surely lead to rational ways of preventing and treating this fearful disability.

*Incontinence*

Ah, now we reach the proper province of the geriatrician. This is something by which he *can* be identified. He is an acknowledged expert in incontinence. He is the chap who knows all about pads and commodes and things. Let us ask him to help us.

To the practitioners of geriatric medicine have been gifted the organs of malodorous malfunction, the lower reaches of the gastro-intestinal and urogenital tracts. Give the chaps a bit of territory they can call their own and keep them quiet.

A slanderous stereotype indeed, and not to be taken too seriously. But how does the specialist in human ageing view his role in these unpleasant parts?

At a time of great improvements in the techniques of waste disposal, the methods of human elimination seem anachronistic and objectionable. A person living to the age of 75 has emptied his bladder approximately 175,000 times successfully, but all is lost the first time the bladder fails. His social valuation and his medical categorisation abruptly change. He is like the solvent who becomes bankrupt: the erstwhile friends to whom he applies for help turn away. Doctors interested in failure of his oesophageal sphincter turn away from his anal sphincter. Those fascinated by incompetence of his mitral valve are turned off by incompetence of his urethral valve, yet the mechanics are no less delicate and failure no less disabling.

Recent developments have put into the hands of the geriatric team techniques for neurophysiological study of the incontinent.[13] Major problems remain in acquiring the diagnostic resources, and in relating the findings to the medical, social and psychological variables forming the backcloth against which the drama of human continence is enacted.

### *Intellectual Impairment*

The brain presides over the liberty of our bodies as Parliament presides over the liberty of our citizens. The brain confers on each muscle its freedom of action, and receives from each sense organ its assessment of the consequence. The failure of a human brain in late life destroys the integrity of the personality and relations between those dear to one another. This ultimate catastrophe of old age was until recently not even accorded the dignity of an objective name – brain failure; but was identified by the pejorative term of senility.[14] Compared with the wealth of effort poured for many years into the investigation of heart failure, the scientific study of brain failure has barely commenced; although the last decade has been extremely fruitful.[15] Where the naive observer may still see only 'confusion', the informed one might spend a clinical lifetime observing the pattern of loss and compensation which characterises brain failure. Few conditions demonstrate better the contrast between prevalence and severity on the one hand and the investment of scientific effort on the other.

## The Quest for Science

'All science', said Lord Kelvin 'is measurement.' Twentieth-century medicine applauds this definition and measures whatever can be inserted into a test tube and much that cannot. The comparative lack of measurement which characterises geriatric medicine as practised in the United Kingdom today is due not to the inherent nature of the speciality but to the want of leisure of those facing the clinical problems and the want of insight of those with scientific equipment.

The giants of geriatrics are measurable but the available instruments are not always appropriate. You can no more measure brain function with a CAT scan than you can measure Mozart with an audiometer. But you can measure those aspects of brain function which you hope to influence by treatment; and the same goes for the functions of muscles, joints, balance, bladder and bowel.

The clinical problems which ill old people present to medical science are at least as enticing and challenging a field of exploration as any conventional speciality. Geriatric medicine has not acquired universal recognition as a speciality not because it lacks potential scientific content but because it lacks recruits.

## The Choice

There are three main patterns of care for the elderly ill, which I would call 'inclusive', 'exclusive' and 'inconclusive' respectively:

(1) a separate service for long-term hospitalisation of old people based on the nursing home principle, with planned admission of selected cases from a waiting list, high quality of in-patient care, and no urge to discharge;
(2) control of all hospital medical admissions by general physicians in high-turnover units, with separate organisation of specialist domiciliary services by non-hospital-based community physicians;
(3) the British system of specialist geriatricians operating an indefinable service to an undefined population in uneasy competition with general physicians who claim the possession of similar skills and resources.

It is my belief that only the third of these models is capable of evolving into the true specialism of human ageing for which I would write the following recipe.

## A Job Description

My job description for the future geriatrician remains firmly based on the British model, with the routine work-load halved, and the opportunity added to specialise in the medical science of human ageing. In my scheme the geriatrician is a member of a team of four consultants, with supporting junior medical staff, who provide an integrated hospital and community service for a population of 250,000. The junior staff rotate with general medical firms. The team has 250 beds divided between not more than two general hospitals. There are 50 day hospital places, and one new out-patient clinic per week for each consultant. The consultant sees patients on request in medical, surgical, orthopaedic and psychiatric units serving the same population, as well as those at home referred to him by the general practitioner. He is in direct charge of both a domiciliary and a hospital-based comprehensive rehabilitation service. A social worker on his staff is closely linked with the provision of these services. In his district there is a terminal care unit with a domiciliary service. He has links with psychiatric services as well.

In addition to the usual range of medical investigation and specialty advice to which his patients have full and equal access, he or one of his colleagues has the following facilities, in collaboration with the appropriate specialist:

(1) a gait laboratory for scientific measurement of gait parameters and monitoring of gait performance. This is used also for the rehabilitation of stroke patients and amputees and there is collaboration with orthopaedic surgeons, rheumatologists and rehabilitation specialists;
(2) a clinic for the investigation of bladder function with urodynamic equipment and an incontinence nurse adviser for assistance in the community;
(3) a clinical psychologist with interest in behaviour modification;
(4) specialist clinics in the neurology, cardiology and rheumatology of old age.

He also has extensive undergraduate and postgraduate teaching and research sessions.

I hope I shall live to see this put into general widespread practice.

## Conclusion

Human ageing is an awesome spectacle. It may be seen only as a time of degradation and decrepitude; or as the astronomer sees the eclipse, as the animal breeder sees the Maverick, as the seismologist sees the earthquake: a natural phenomenon, fearful in its beauty and in its revelation of nature – an opportunity for the advancement of science and of human knowledge. For the doctor it affords an unrivalled opportunity for the provision of a satisfying medical service that restores some health and happiness to the later years and that provides some recognition and respect for those who have lived long.

Is geriatric medicine a specialty? Yes, emphatically, it is the specialty of human ageing.

## References


1. Parkhouse, J., Palmer, M.K., and Hambleton, B.A. (1979) 'Career Preferences of Doctors Qualifying in the United Kingdom in 1977', *Health Trends, 11*, 38-41
2. Bourne, S., and Bruggen, P. (1978) 'Re-examination of the Distinction Award System in England and Wales, 1976: the New Advisory Committees', *Brit. Med. J., 1*, 456-8
3. McArdle, C., Wylie, J.C., and Alexander, W.P. (1975) 'Geriatric Patients in Acute Medical Wards', *Brit. Med. J., 4*, 568-70
4. Adams, G.F. (1974) 'Eld health', *Brit. Med. J., 7*, 789-91
5. Royal College of Physicians (1977) *Medical Care of the Elderly: Report of the Working Party of the Royal College of Physicians of London', Lancet, 1*, 1092-5
6. Bagnall, W.E., Datta, S.R., Knox, J., and Horrocks, P. (1977) 'Geriatric Medicine in Hull: a Comprehensive Review', *Brit. Med. J., 2*, 102-4
7. Department of Health and Social Security (1976) *Priorities for Health and and Personal Social Services in England*, HMSO, London
8. Isaacs, B., Livingstone, M., and Neville, Y. (1972) *Survival of the Unfittest*, Routledge and Kegan Paul, London
9. Isaacs, B. (1976) *The Giants of Geriatrics*, Inaugural lecture, University of Birmingham
10. Paul, J.P. (1974) 'Comparison of EMG Signals from Leg Muscles with the Corresponding Force Actions Calculated from Walkpath Measurements' in *Human Locomotor Engineering*, Institute of Mechanical Engineers, London, pp. 16-26
11. Roberts, T.D.M. (1978) *Neurophysiology of Postural Mechanisms*, 2nd edn, Butterworths, London
12. Herman, R. (ed.) (1976) *Neural Control of Locomotion. Advances in Behavioural Biology, vol. 18,* Plenum Press, New York
13. Caldwell, K.P.S. (1975) (ed.) *Urinary Incontinence,* Sector Publishing, London
14. Isaacs, B., and Caird, F.I. (1976) '"Brain Failure": a Contribution to the Terminology of Mental Abnormality in Old Age', *Age and Ageing, 5*, 241-4
15. Ordy, J.M., and Brizzee, K.R. (1975) *Neurology of Ageing, an Inter-disciplinary Life-span Approach. Advances in Behavioural Biology, vol. 16*, Plenum Press, New York

# CONTRIBUTORS

Tom Arie, Professor of Health Care of the Elderly, University of Nottingham, England.

Klaus Bergmann, Physician, The Bethlem Royal Hospital and The Maudsley Hospital, London, England.

Roy V. Boyd, Physician, Department of Health Care of the Elderly, Sherwood Hospital, Nottingham, England.

Donald B. Calne, Clinical Director, National Institute of Neurological and Communicative Disorders and Stroke, Bethesda, Maryland, USA

J. Grimley Evans, Professor of Medicine (Geriatrics), University of Newcastle-upon-Tyne, England.

A. Norman Exton-Smith, Barlow Professor of Geriatric Medicine, University College Hospital Medical School, London, England.

Bernard Isaacs, Charles Hayward Professor of Geriatric Medicine, University of Birmingham, England.

David Jolley, Psychogeriatrician, Withington Hospital, Manchester, England; Hon. Lecturer, University of Manchester.

Graham Mulley, Physician, Department of Health Care of the Elderly, Sherwood Hospital, Nottingham, England.

Felix Post, Physician Emeritus, The Bethlem Royal Hospital and The Maudsley Hospital, London, England.

Kenneth Shulman, Psychiatrist, Sunnybrook Hospital, Toronto, Ontario, Canada; Assistant Professor, University of Toronto.

Olive Stevenson, Professor of Social Policy and Social Work, University of Keele, England.

Adrian Verwoerdt, Professor of Psychiatry, Duke University Medical Center, Durham, North Carolina, USA.

James Williamson, Professor of Geriatric Medicine, University of Edinburgh, Scotland.

# INDEX

For Product Safety Concerns and Information please contact our EU representative GPSR@taylorandfrancis.com Taylor & Francis Verlag GmbH, Kaufingerstraße 24, 80331 München, Germany